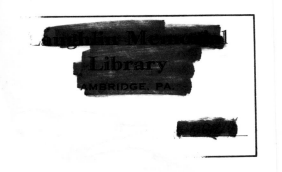

Drugs and Sports

by Don Nardo

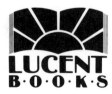

LUCENT
B·O·O·K·S

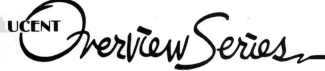

Look for these and other books in the Lucent Overview series:

Acid Rain
AIDS
Animal Rights
The Beginning of Writing
Dealing with Death
Drug Trafficking
Drugs and Sports
Endangered Species

Energy Alternatives
Garbage
Homeless Children
Smoking
Special Effects in the Movies
Teen Alcoholism
The UFO Challenge
Vietnam

Library of Congress Cataloging-in-Publication Data

Nardo, Don, 1947-
  Drugs and sports / by Don Nardo.
    p. cm. — (Overview series)
  Includes bibliographical references
   ISBN 1-56006-112-X
    1. Doping in sports. I. Title. II. Series: Lucent overview
series.
RC1230.N37 1990
362.29'088796—dc20   90-6686
                                                                           CIP
                                                                            AC

*To Bill, who learned the hard way that
wrestlers make rotten basketball players.*

Contents

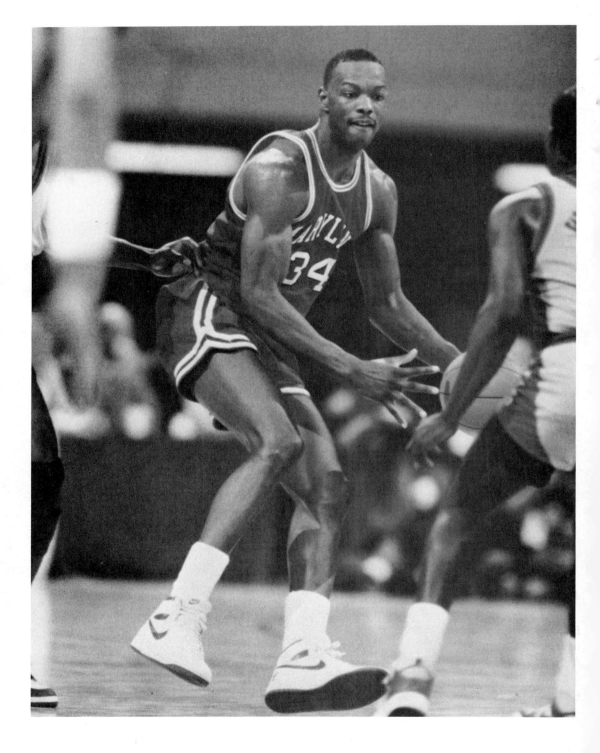

1

Athletes and Addiction

GREEK MYTHOLOGY tells of a young god named Morpheus. He was the god of dreams and the son of Hypnos, the god of sleep. In the land of Libya, where summer lasted all year long, Morpheus planted a special purple flower called the lotus. Soon the people of that land smelled the sweet flowers and ate them. They immediately fell into a deep, untroubled sleep. From that day on, they awoke only long enough to gather the lotus flowers; then they ate the flowers and slept once again.

When the Greek king Ulysses and his men visited Libya, or Lotusland, some of the strong, athletic sailors ate the flowers. The men quickly became addicted to the drug in the flowers. They lost their strength and willpower and wanted only to drift in and out of the pleasant sleep. Ulysses had to drag his men back to the ship and chain them until the effects of the drug had worn off.

The story of the lotus-eaters and similar tales from ancient times show us that drug use is not new. People have faced drug problems all through the ages. Today, these problems threaten all members of society, even those people who do not use drugs. For example, law enforcement experts estimate that

Basketball star Len Bias moves down the court with the ball. Bias, who played for the University of Maryland, died of a cocaine overdose in 1986.

more than half of all violent crimes reported in the United States in the last few years have been drug-related. Robberies and break-ins are committed by people who need money to support their drug habits. Washington, D.C., the nation's capital, is sometimes referred to as the nation's "murder capital" because of its unusually high rate of drug-related killings.

Each year, thousands of tons of illegal drugs are smuggled into the United States. Federal, state, and local officials spend billions of dollars trying to stop these drugs from entering the country. But the officials say that the scale of illegal drug trafficking is so huge that they are able to seize only a small fraction of the incoming flow.

Legal vs. illegal drugs

Of course, not all drugs are illegal. Over the centuries, doctors have learned to harness the powers of some drugs to kill pain and help heal the sick. Most societies have recognized that, in the hands of a doctor, drugs can be useful. Such medicinal use of drugs has been and continues to be legal and accepted.

But the same drugs used by doctors can often be *mis*used by others. An example is cocaine, which was initially used by doctors for numbing pain. Cocaine later came to be used illegally by large numbers of people and is highly addictive. Drug officials claim that a majority of drug-related crimes involve some form of cocaine.

When drugs such as cocaine are used for pleasure or personal satisfaction, they are called recreational drugs. Marijuana, derived from the hemp plant, is another illegal recreational drug that is widely used. But not all recreational drugs are illegal. For instance, the two most often used recreational drugs—alcohol and nicotine (found in tobacco) —are legal. Like cocaine, alcohol and nicotine are

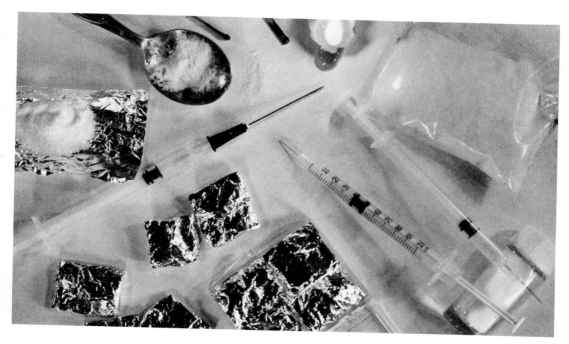

highly addictive. Also, both produce serious health problems and are responsible for over 500,000 deaths each year. Yet use of these drugs has been accepted by modern society.

Drugs and the athlete

Recreational drugs, both legal and illegal, are used by members of every social group. They are used by young and old, by rich and poor, and by members of every race and religious group. Athletes are no exception, and drug use in the sports world is widespread.

It should be understood that not all athletes misuse drugs. Many do not take them at all. But the problem of drug abuse by athletes has grown to such proportions in recent years that it has become a matter of international concern.

According to Rick Reilly, a writer for *Sports Illustrated*, the use of drugs by athletes has become a major problem: "Not that drug abuse is anything

Illegal drugs, such as cocaine and heroin, are smuggled into the United States each year. Shown with the drugs are the items employed in their illegal use.

new in sports; it has just picked up a terrible new momentum," said Reilly.

Recreational drugs, however, are not the only chemical substances used by athletes. Sports involve physical performance, and athletes have always sought ways to improve that performance. Sometimes they have resorted to using drugs. Substances used to improve strength, speed, or personal image are referred to as performance-enhancing drugs.

The use of performance-enhancing drugs is not a recent development. Centuries ago, for instance, the Kaffir people of South Africa drank a substance called *dop* before competing in sporting events or fighting in battle. The Kaffir believed that *dop*, a mixture of alcohol and cola, gave them the extra energy they needed to win. Later, the Europeans who settled in South Africa added an *e* to the word, and *dope* became a term applied to all drugs.

A history of athlete drug use

There were other early experiments with drugs to improve performance. In the 1800s, athletes tried swallowing concentrated doses of caffeine (a stimulant found in coffee) or sugar cubes coated with ether (an anesthetic used in operations). Some runners tried consuming nitroglycerin, a powerful chemical prescribed by doctors to relieve heart pain. The runners thought the drug would make their hearts pump blood, but it only gave them bad headaches. Other athletes swallowed mixtures of cocaine and heroin or deadly poisons like strychnine. Recently, steroids have become the most common performance-enhancing drugs and are taken to increase physical strength and body size. Steroid use solely for the purpose of increasing strength is illegal in some states. A doctor's prescription is required to obtain the drug in all states.

While some use of recreational and performance-enhancing drugs in sports has been known for generations, the users have generally constituted a small minority of athletes. Therefore, for a long time, the use of drugs by athletes did not appear to be a problem. Beginning in the 1950s, however, drug use by athletes began to increase. In the 1960s, heroin addiction claimed the lives of several football players, including the popular "Big Daddy" Lipscomb of the Baltimore Colts. In the 1970s, baseball player Dock Ellis was found to be pitching under the influence of the hallucinogen LSD.

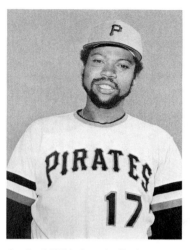

In the 1970s, baseball player Dock Ellis was found to be under the influence of LSD while pitching.

By the 1980s, drug use in sports was described by experts, including Dr. William N. Taylor, formerly with the U.S. Olympic Drug Control Program, as an "epidemic." In 1986, the untimely death of basketball star Len Bias called more attention to the problem. Bias, who played for the University of Maryland, died of a cocaine overdose. People throughout the country were shocked and saddened. Bias had been intelligent and talented, with what appeared to be a bright future ahead of him.

Referring to Bias's death, the Reverend Jesse Jackson said, "On a day the children mourn, I hope they learn." Unfortunately, many athletes did not learn. Eight days after Bias died, Don Rogers, a safety for the Cleveland Browns, also lost his life as the result of a cocaine overdose. Three days after that, Willie Smith, also of the Browns, was arrested on cocaine and weapons charges.

A drastic increase in steroid use

Along with the increase in the use of recreational drugs, the use of performance-enhancing drugs also increased from the 1950s to the 1980s. By the mid-1980s, some players in the National Football League (NFL) claimed that at least 40 percent of the players in the league were using illegal steroids.

Others placed the figure at 70 percent or even higher. In general, drug-related arrests by police or suspensions by team officials became more common in the world of team sports.

But the drugs-in-sports epidemic encompasses more than just illegal drugs. Use of legal drugs like alcohol has also increased in recent years among athletes. Though some famous baseball players of the past, such as Babe Ruth and Mickey Mantle, were known to abuse alcohol, most people saw them as exceptions. More recent baseball stars like Sam McDowell and Bob Welch admitted to being alcoholics. They also said they were not exceptions and that abuse of alcohol had become widespread in their sport, even on the high school level.

Drug abuse affects everyone

It is possible that a link exists between drug abuse in sports and drug abuse in society as a whole. Because sports is such an important and

Many people do not consider alcohol a drug, because it is legal and accepted in society. However, alcohol abuse can have a negative effect on athletic performance.

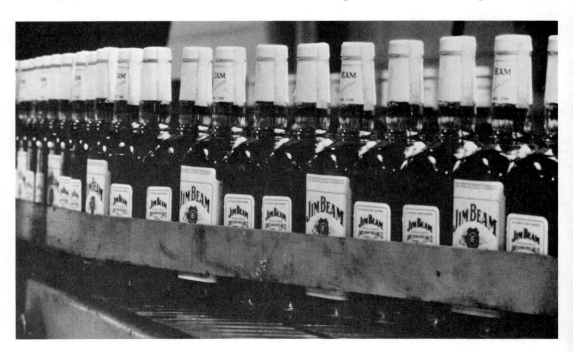

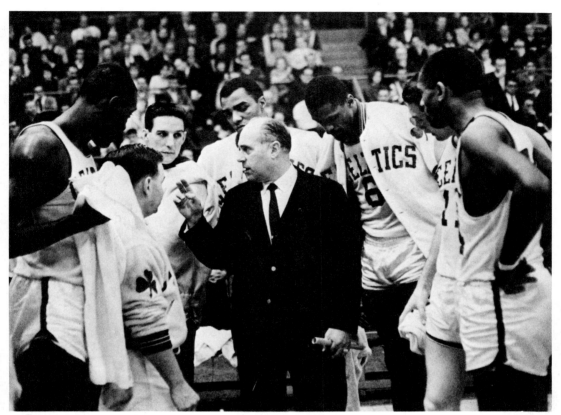

popular institution in the United States, what famous athletes do can have an effect on what non-athletes do. Fans tend to mimic the actions of their sports heroes, including using drugs. Therefore, an increase in drug use by professional athletes can result in an increase in drug use in society overall.

The use of drugs by athletes can also help popularize the drugs. It is almost as if the athletes were advertising the drugs, making it easier for drug dealers to sell their products. "Drug people aren't stupid. They know that if they can addict a superstar . . . they can link themselves to his name, to his fame. Then they can get other people to fall in line a little easier," said Red Auerbach, president of the Boston Celtics.

Players gather around Arnold "Red" Auerbach, the Boston Celtics coach and general manager. Auerbach maintains that drug abuse by famous athletes spurs abuse in the general public.

Other people argue that the situation works in reverse, that what happens in society affects what athletes do. They think more athletes are taking drugs because drug use in all areas of society is increasing. In other words, the more drugs are used and accepted by the general population, the more athletes will use drugs, since athletes are members of the general population.

Why athletes take drugs

The reasons athletes themselves give for taking drugs are varied. Some cite peer pressure. If a lot of people on a team are using a drug, other members of the team might take the drug to fit in. Some players claim to use recreational drugs to relax and relieve the stress caused by training and competition. And many athletes take drugs to improve their performance.

There are also those athletes who experiment with drugs for fun. These players are usually young and see themselves as invincible, both on and off the playing field. They are convinced that no drug can hook them. But the tragedies of Len Bias, Don Rogers, and hundreds of others like them prove that no one is immune to the dangers.

The stories of athletes being harmed by drug use recall the tale of Ulysses's band of athlete-warriors and their troubles with the lotus flowers. For many sports figures, the world of drug use has become the modern version of Lotusland. Whether or not the link between the worlds of drugs and sports will continue will depend on many factors, including education, public opinion, and the attitudes of individual athletes.

Sports-drug issues being hotly debated range from the fairness of drug testing to whether steroid use should be allowed in sports. There are impressive arguments on both sides of each issue, and most people agree that these questions have no easy answers. Perhaps that is because the use of drugs by athletes is so deeply rooted in both the past and present of human experience. Indeed, the topic of drugs and sports is as old as humanity itself and as new as tomorrow morning's newspaper headlines.

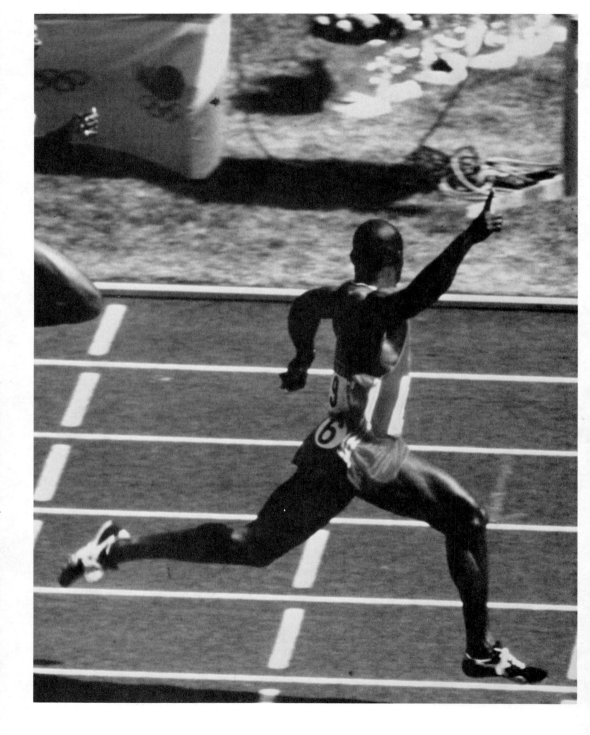

2

Steroids: Hercules in a Bottle

IT WAS TIME for the one hundred-meter dash at the 1988 summer Olympics in Seoul, South Korea. Canadian track star Ben Johnson, who already held the world record of 9.83 seconds, left the starting blocks and never looked back. Johnson thrilled the world, setting a new world and Olympic record of 9.79 seconds. But Johnson's moment of victory was short-lived. Only sixty-nine hours later, the International Olympic Committee (IOC), which banned the use of steroids in 1973, announced the results of its routine drug testing of all competing athletes. Johnson had tested positive for stanozolol, a steroid used by many athletes to increase muscle strength (which contributes to speed).

Johnson was disqualified and disgraced. His gold medal was taken away and awarded to Carl Lewis, the American runner who had placed second in the race. Later, the International Amateur Athletic Federation (IAAF) suspended Johnson from competing for two years.

Ben Johnson's use of steroids was far from being an isolated case. An article by Michael Janofsky for *The New York Times* stated that medical and legal experts as well as drug traffickers estimated that at least half of the nine thousand athletes who competed at the Seoul Olympics had used steroids to train.

Canadian track star Ben Johnson wins a gold medal in the 1988 summer Olympics in Seoul, South Korea. Sixty-nine hours later, Johnson was forced to relinquish his medal after he tested positive for steroids.

17

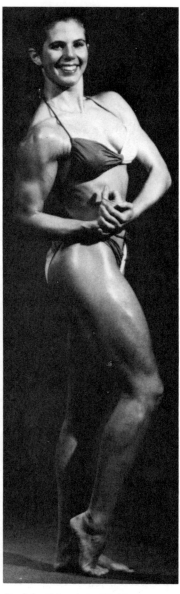

Bodybuilder Amy Goldwater poses for the camera. Although Goldwater does not use steroids, some bodybuilders maintain that the use of steroids to promote muscle growth is widespread in this sport.

The 1988 Olympics shares the humiliation of steroid abuse with Olympics of the past. At the World Class track and field meet in Zurich, Switzerland, in 1987, as many as fourteen athletes did not participate in their events after testing positive for steroids. Earlier, at Caracas, Venezuela, in 1983, fifteen athletes who had taken steroids were not allowed to compete.

In addition, dozens of American college football players have been barred from playing in bowl games because they took steroids. One professional football player said that more than 75 percent of all athletes are now using steroids. And some competitive bodybuilders claim that steroids are used by nearly 100 percent of those who participate in their sport.

Steroid use is widespread

Steroid use is not limited to professional or amateur athletics. Nor is it restricted to any particular sport. Bodybuilders, football players, baseball players, runners, and swimmers use steroids. And even though steroids have been banned by sports groups such as the National Football League (NFL), the National Collegiate Athletic Association (NCAA), and the U.S. Powerlifting Federation (USPF), many athletes continue to take them. "An estimated one million U.S. athletes are taking steroids," said Marty Duda, editor for the *Physician and Sports Medicine* magazine.

Men are not the only users of steroids. More and more women are turning to steroids to give them an edge over other athletes. Olympic sprinter Evelyn Ashford said that the use of steroids is becoming more prevalent among women in track and field. And Pat Connolly, a former Olympian, said she believes that as many as twenty women in the 1988 Seoul Olympics had trained with steroids.

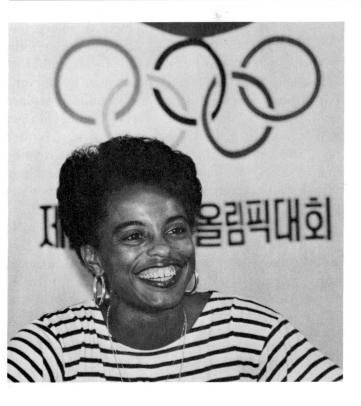

During the 1988 summer Olympics, a smiling U.S. track and field star Evelyn Ashford answers questions during a press conference. Ashford believes steroid use is increasing among women in track and field.

What exactly is this drug that is so widely used by athletes, often at the risk of their health as well as suspensions and public humiliation? Steroids are powerful chemicals that are similar to testosterone, a male hormone. A hormone is a substance produced in living cells that affects or stimulates other body cells in various ways. For example, some hormones stimulate growth. Testosterone maintains secondary sexual characteristics in men, such as a deep voice, facial hair, and aggressive behavior. Since steroids are similar to testosterone, they can also produce these characteristics. In addition, steroids promote the growth of muscle tissue; anabolic steroids is the term for these substances that build up body tissue.

Steroids can be natural or artificial, and there are dozens of different versions of the drug.

Steroids have two basic uses: medical and performance-enhancing. In the field of medicine, steroids have been found to be effective in a number of areas, and are often legally prescribed by doctors. For instance, doctors use certain steroids to replace testosterone in men and boys whose bodies do not make enough of the hormone. The drug has also been effective in healing injuries as well as treating malnutrition, problems with bones, and some blood disorders. Sometimes, doctors use steroids to offset the harsh effects of cancer radiation treatments.

As a performance-enhancing drug, anabolic steroids have sometimes been shown to produce small increases in body weight and muscle mass. Muscle mass is directly related to strength. Generally speaking, the bigger the muscle, the

A physical therapist bandages an athlete's injury before a game. Some doctors prescribe steroids to heal sports-related injuries.

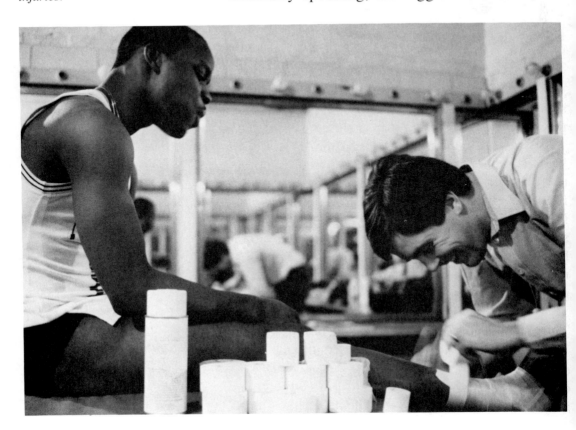

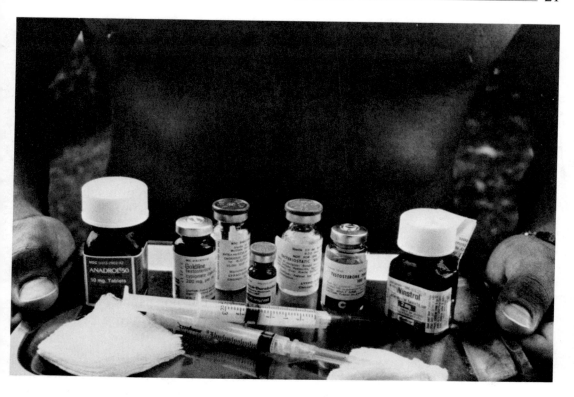

stronger it is. Therefore, steroids are most often used by athletes as strength-building aids.

To obtain steroids, hundreds of thousands of athletes resort to illegal methods. Some forge prescriptions. Others buy the substance "under the counter" from druggists looking to make some easy money. Most illegal steroids are ordered through the mail or sold to athletes by dealers who make the rounds of health clubs, gyms, and high schools. Experts estimate that the steroid black market now tops $100 million per year in sales.

An athlete displays some of the many different versions of steroids. This drug can be natural or artificial, and is used for medical reasons or to enhance performance and appearance.

The physical effects of steroids

Several studies and experiments have been conducted in recent years on steroids and their effects on animals and humans. The findings of these studies have not always been consistent. But most have

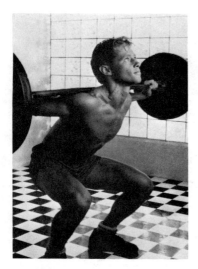

A bodybuilder performs squats while pumping iron. Other athletes in this sport have been accused of using steroids to increase muscle tissue, because larger muscles increase the athlete's capacity to lift heavy weights.

shown that small doses of steroids do indeed increase muscle mass and strength. The drug also slightly reduces body fat in those who take it regularly. These are the beneficial effects of steroids.

Harmful effects of steroids

Several negative effects of steroids, however, have also been repeatedly observed. For example, the drug causes liver problems in some people. One job the liver does is break down drugs that enter the body. Large amounts of steroids might overload the organ and lead to liver damage. If the liver is not working correctly, jaundice, a yellowing of the skin and whites of the eyes, can occur. In this condition, toxic substances can leak into the bloodstream. Jaundice is serious but not usually fatal, and the condition can be reversed when a person stops taking steroids.

Steroids can also cause blood-filled cysts to form in the liver. These cysts can rupture and cause the liver to stop working. In addition, some people who have been treated medically with steroids have developed liver tumors. Most of these were not dangerous, but some cancerous, or malignant, tumors have been found. One male bodybuilder who had regularly consumed anabolic steroids died from such a tumor.

Steroids also appear to adversely affect the cardiovascular system, which includes the heart and arteries. With prolonged steroid use, a person may experience a lowering of levels of high-density lipoproteins (HDL), the "good" cholesterol manufactured by the body (cholesterol is a fatty substance present in all animals, including people). Since HDL helps get rid of "bad" cholesterol, lowering the HDL level can cause the bad version to build up slowly in a regular steroid user. The results can be increases in blood pressure and eventually a heart attack or stroke.

Also, experiments with animals have indicated that steroids can damage the heart muscle itself. Once a person stops taking the drug, such damage can usually be reversed. But it is possible that the heart may be damaged beyond repair. In this case, a heart transplant is the only way to save the patient's life.

Steroids damaging effects

There are several effects of steroids on the reproductive system. In the body, this is the system responsible for sexual function and producing children. Steroids can reduce sperm production in males, making it difficult or impossible for a man to father children. In addition, steroids seem to lower the amount of sex hormones a man naturally produces, which then reduces his interest in sex. As with the cardiovascular system, a man's reproductive system will return to normal after steroids have been eliminated from the body. But the recovery process can take many months.

In women, as in men, steroid use has been shown to lower the production of sex hormones, again reducing interest in sex. Also, steroids can cause fewer eggs to develop, making it more difficult for pregnancy to occur. In addition, a woman taking steroids can undergo physical changes associated with the male sex hormone testosterone. She can develop facial hair, a deepening of the voice, reduction of breast size, and episodes of unusually aggressive behavior. In the cases of some women, the secondary sex characteristics did not go away after they ceased taking the drug.

Steroids also have psychological or emotional effects on people who use them. Users often experience mood swings. They can go from feeling happy to feeling angry or depressed in only a few seconds. Researchers have also noticed changes in brain

A bodybuilder lifting hand weights is an example of a female athlete who does not have to use steroids to maintain a muscular physique. Some female bodybuilders use steroids to increase muscle size, strength, shape, and definition. Females taking steroids may develop secondary sex characteristics, such as a deepening of the voice.

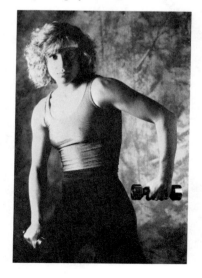

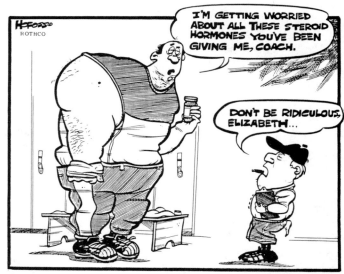

© Hofoss/Rothco

wave activity in steroid users. These changes are similar to those observed after a person uses stimulants or antidepressants.

The aggressive, sometimes hostile behavior associated with steroids is often seen as a desirable effect by athletes who use the drug. For instance, some football players using steroids describe their increased desire to "destroy" their opponents and win games. Weight lifters tell how the drug helps them get "psyched up" to see the barbell as an enemy to be overcome. While such a hostile mental attitude might be useful on the playing field or in the gym, it is undesirable, even dangerous in everyday life.

Sometimes the steroid-induced hostility of athletes spills over into the nonathletic world and affects innocent people. For example, several police officers who used steroids while weight lifting off duty were recently suspended or fired from their jobs. The steroids made the officers' behavior so aggressive that the men verbally or physically abused citizens they were supposed to be helping.

In one incident, a female shopkeeper complained to an officer about the police using her phone too much. The man flew into a rage, pulled out his gun, and shot the woman. She is now in a wheelchair and paralyzed for life.

Who uses steroids and why?

Most of the athletes using steroids are those who participate in sports where strength is a major factor. Weight lifters and bodybuilders, for example, are often considered to be the most common steroid abusers. These athletes have learned exactly which steroids to use to achieve specific goals. Dianabol, for instance, is a steroid used by lifters to build muscle size and strength. Anavar and maxibloin, on the other hand, are steroids that bodybuilders feel give their muscles the appearance of hardness. Still another steroid, primobolin, is said to add definition, or shape, to the muscles.

These and many other steroids have been listed in

A weight lifter pauses during the 1988 summer Olympics. Weight lifters such as this one, who do not use steroids, claim that it is difficult to compete with opponents who use the drug.

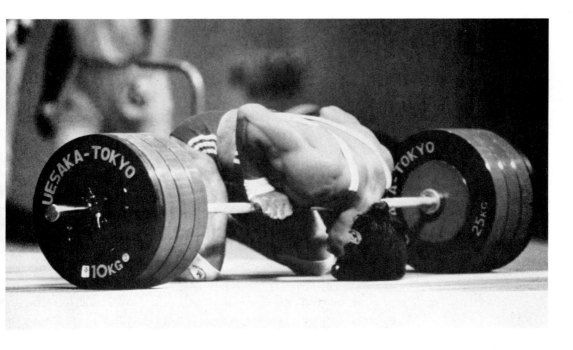

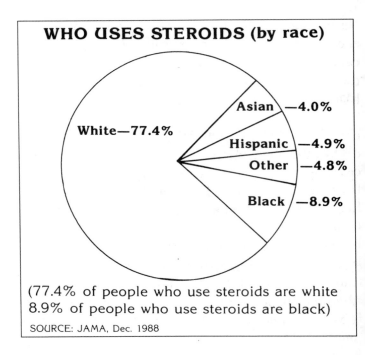

WHO USES STEROIDS (by race)

White—77.4%

Asian—4.0%

Hispanic—4.9%

Other—4.8%

Black—8.9%

(77.4% of people who use steroids are white
8.9% of people who use steroids are black)

SOURCE: JAMA, Dec. 1988

a controversial eighteen-page pamphlet titled *The Underground Steroid Handbook*. The author is former bodybuilder Dan Duchaine, who refers to himself as a "steroids consultant." Others have called him a steroids "guru." Describing his knowledge of steroids, Duchaine says, "I'm the only person to combine technical information from research study, anecdotal information from around the world, and hands-on experience with human lab rats, including myself."

Duchaine disagrees with doctors and medical studies that claim steroids are always dangerous. "You cannot accept for a fact that steroids have harmful side effects," insists Duchaine. "Some are more dangerous than others; some are not dangerous at all." Basically, Duchaine believes that steroids are safe if used in small, controlled amounts. The steroid guru has had a definite influence on athletes in the sport of bodybuilding, including at least one

Mr. Universe. Duchaine himself believes his influence has been positive. Many members of the medical community, however, see him as a promoter of dangerous substances—drugs that are potentially harmful to athletes and nonathletes alike.

In addition to weight lifters and bodybuilders, other athletes, such as wrestlers, shot-putters, and discus throwers, also rely on physical power to compete. Not surprisingly, steroids are heavily used by athletes in these sports as well. Many sprinters, like Ben Johnson, have used steroids to increase their speed. Since a runner's speed is directly related to the strength in his or her leg muscles, the use of steroids seems to promise a faster race. More and more runners, fearing they cannot compete against opponents using the drug, are giving in and taking steroids during training.

A sprinter takes off for the finish line. Although this athlete does not use steroids, some sprinters use the drug to increase muscle mass, because strength of leg muscles is a main factor in running speed.

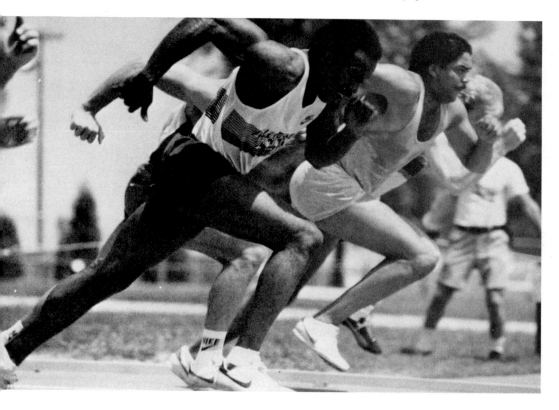

Football is a sport that demands a combination of both unusual strength and speed. The use of steroids in football now seems to be the rule rather than the exception. With so many players taking the drug, more and more athletes are experiencing its negative effects, physically and otherwise. Consider the case of Brian Bosworth, who was an all-American linebacker for the University of Oklahoma. Bosworth was barred from playing in the 1987 Orange Bowl because he tested positive for steroids. He claimed to have taken the drug to help heal injuries. Like Duchaine, Bosworth does not see steroids as a major drug threat, and he resents the treatment he received by football officials. "I'll continue to fight against the use of drugs—recreational drugs that are destroying society. Steroids aren't destroying society," Bosworth said.

The benefits of steroid use

Steve Courson is one athlete who would disagree with Bosworth. Courson once played offensive guard for the Tampa Bay Buccaneers. Like many other NFL players, he regularly took steroids to "bulk up" and increase his strength. Courson knew that steroids could be dangerous, but he believed the benefits outweighed the drawbacks. "In order to compete in this business, you absolutely have to know the pluses and minuses that come along with using steroids," Courson said. Eventually, Courson changed his mind about using steroids. In 1985, after nine years in pro football, Courson had to retire because of problems with his heart. His heart rate, without exertion, was a dangerously rapid 150 beats per minute. Courson believes that his ailment is related to his prolonged use of steroids. Describing his condition, his doctor said, "Steve's heart is stretched and dilated. It is flabby and baggy and doesn't pump as a normal heart should." Experts agree that Courson's best chance for recov-

In 1987, linebacker Brian Bosworth tested positive for steroids and was barred from playing in the Orange Bowl. Bosworth claims that he was taking the drug for an injury and believes steroids are safe in small amounts.

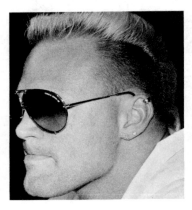

ery is a heart transplant.

Courson's case was one of several that prompted the NFL to strengthen its antisteroid policy. At first, the league had no official rules for dealing with steroid users. But as of 1989, those players who test positive for steroids get a thirty-day suspension for the first offense. For a second offense, the player is suspended for the season. But Courson and others have pointed out that the tests can be beaten. If a player knows a test is coming up, he can stop taking the drug in time to get it out of his system before the test. After the test, he can go right back to taking steroids.

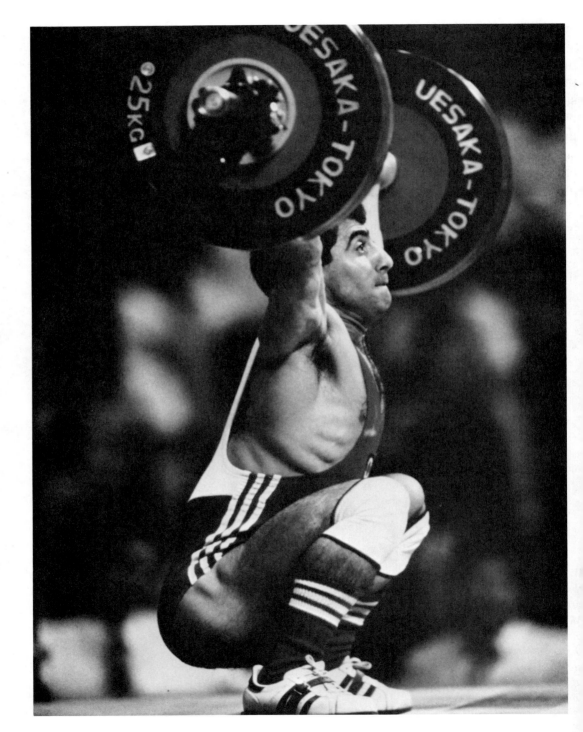

Steroids: A Muscular Controversy

STEVE COURSON feels his career and perhaps his entire life was wrecked by using steroids. Because of the pain the drug has caused him, Courson hopes to see younger athletes become fearful of taking steroids. He and many other sports figures are alarmed at the increasing use of the drug by college and high school athletes. The popular nicknames for the drug—"roid," "gas," and "juice"—are heard in college and high school locker rooms.

Joseph Biden Jr., chairman of the Senate Judiciary Committee, cites a study that warns of the dangers that threaten the more than 500,000 young athletes who use steroids: "Steroid use permeates all levels of sports, threatening the futures of hundreds of thousands of teenagers," said Biden.

People who are against steroid use point out that young athletes have no idea what they are getting into when they begin to use the drug. "I wish I could be seventeen again and know what I know now," says Fletcher McLane Jr., a former Wisconsin college football player. "I lost everything except my life."

Weight lifter Oxen Mirzoian of he USSR demonstrates his great strength. Although Mirzoian does not use steroids, other weight lifters claim that he psychological effects of teroids, such as hostility and aggression, are beneficial during competition.

McLane began as a 165-pound high school quarterback. Steroids transformed him into a 275-pounder with a neck one observer likened to a tree trunk. McLane's face became covered with acne scars, and boils broke out on his arms and legs. Acne and boils are frequent side effects of steroid use. The young man developed high blood pressure. He became extremely aggressive, repeatedly getting into fights and being thrown out of gyms for breaking equipment. After he flew into a rage and wrecked a section of his dorm, he was expelled from college.

At home, McLane ripped the door off the refrigerator and punched holes in the walls. Still, he continued to increase his dosage of steroids. Finally, he attacked and nearly killed a former teammate. The police arrested McLane. "That's when I realized I had a problem," McLane said later. "I swore I wasn't going to take steroids any more. All it takes is one guy to walk into the gym all blown up, and I start thinking of the roids. It's an addiction. But I'm determined never to go through it again."

Parents and coaches influence steroid use

The problem of steroid use involves not only the athletes but coaches and parents as well. One physical education coordinator described the situation: "Coaches who are looking for bulk and don't know the effects of steroids are recommending them. Parents go along because a coach tells them their kid will be a strapping six-footer and will have a great shot at getting a scholarship." Dr. William N. Taylor, of the U.S. Olympic Drug Control Program, also sees parents as a problem when it comes to steroids: "I have received dozens of calls from fathers who want to make their average-sized children bigger. I've had offers of tens of thousands of dollars to chemically manipulate children."

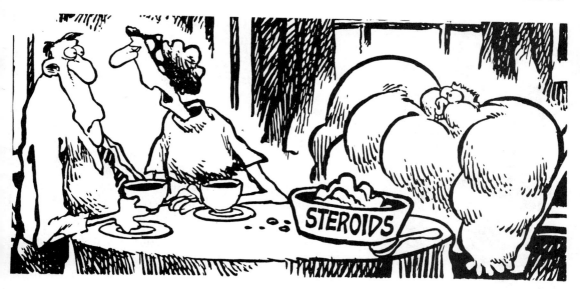

JUNIOR SAYS IT'S THE BREAKFAST OF CHAMPIONS...

Reprinted by permission of UFS, Inc.

Despite the long list of the serious physical and mental effects of steroid use and stories of athletes' ruined lives, there are those, like Dan Duchaine and Brian Bosworth, who maintain that steroids are not the menace so many people claim them to be.

Ron Hale, a former U.S. weight lifting champion, agrees with Duchaine that steroids are perfectly safe when taken in small doses. Hale claims to have taken the drug for more than twenty years without any adverse health problems. "Used properly, they [steroids] are no more of a threat to an adult than liquor is. I've known many people who've used them, and except for one national champion who took very large doses, I don't know anyone who's had trouble," Hale said.

Hale points out that communist countries give steroids to their athletes. He argues that American athletes must take the drug in order to compete as well as their communist opponents. Hale recalls his

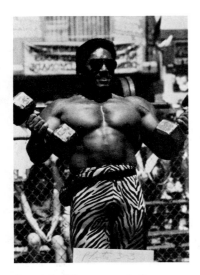

A weight lifter poses before crowds at Muscle Beach in Venice, California.

own athletic record in order to prove steroids help an athlete perform better:

> Even though I was a state champion, I started taking steroids because I thought my progress was slowing. I was five feet, five inches tall and weighed 155 pounds. I could lift a total of 1,150 pounds in the three lifts the event requires. [After using steroids for three years and weighing 165 pounds,] I won the U.S. senior power-lifting title with 1,425 pounds. In all, I've won nine state titles, and I think I'd probably have won most of them without steroids. But there's no way I could have won that national title without them.

Hale also believes that steroid use is an issue of personal freedom. He thinks that people have the right to do whatever they want with their own bodies. He does not think that sports teams or organizations should tell people they cannot use steroids. In addition, he thinks Brian Bosworth's suspension for testing positive for steroids was unfair. Bosworth was taking the drug for an injury. But, says Hale, even if there had not been an injury, it was Bosworth's constitutional right to take steroids. Hale says that steroids do not alter the mind in any way and taking them is not addictive.

According to Hale, the National Collegiate Athletic Association (NCAA) and other sports organizations should stop worrying about athletes taking steroids. Instead, the organizations should concentrate on trying to stop the use of recreational drugs such as marijuana.

Young boys should not use steroids

Hale does caution that his argument applies only to adults. He states that teenagers should never use steroids because the drug stunts growth. He would not let his twelve-year-old son take steroids but feels when the boy is grown, it will be all right for him to do so.

Dan Duchaine and Ron Hale are not the only people in the sports world who argue for the right of athletes to use steroids. Dr. Norman Fost, director of the Program in Medical Ethics at the University of Wisconsin, also thinks that steroids should not be banned. Fost says that he personally does not favor steroid use in sports. He agrees that steroids pose a dangerous threat to an athlete's health. He believes, however, that the arguments for banning steroids are often unreasonable. Fost's complaint focuses on the issue of fairness in athletic competition. He contends that two athletes entering the meet on unequal terms is not necessarily unfair.

Natural advantages

Many athletes, Fost points out, already possess natural advantages over their opponents. This is considered acceptable by players and fans alike. For example, no one argues it is unfair that Robert Parrish of the Boston Celtics is taller than many other basketball players. Similarly, Indianapolis Colts football star Eric Dickerson is not banned

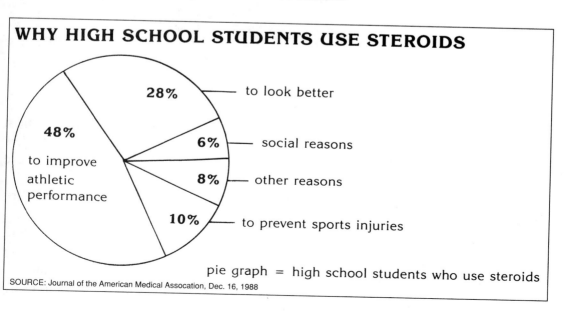

WHY HIGH SCHOOL STUDENTS USE STEROIDS

- 28% — to look better
- 6% — social reasons
- 8% — other reasons
- 10% — to prevent sports injuries
- 48% to improve athletic performance

pie graph = high school students who use steroids

SOURCE: Journal of the American Medical Association, Dec. 16, 1988

In many cases, great strength and speed are not the results of steroid use. Eric Dickerson of the Indianapolis Colts is an example of a super athlete with natural strength and athletic ability.

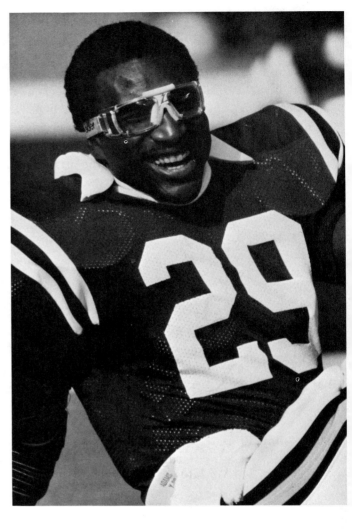

from the field because he is stronger and faster than most other players. These and other super athletes are simply using the bodies and talents they were born with.

Sometimes, the advantage of one athlete over another results from human decision. For instance, consider the hypothetical case of a high school tennis player. She is not necessarily stronger or faster than any of her opponents. However, she puts in twice as many practice hours as they do. As a result, she might defeat them all and win the state championship. She quite clearly walks onto the court with an unequal advantage, namely her extreme dedication. But no one expects officials to cry foul and take back her championship trophy.

Of course, some sports attempt to match opponents evenly. Collegiate wrestlers, for instance, are paired according to weight. Also, men and women do not usually compete against each other. But, in general, most sports allow athletes with natural or other advantages to play against each other.

Many athletes try to enhance their performance by eating special diets (low-fat diets, for instance), according to Fost. They also take daily doses of vitamins and minerals. There is no doubt that such methods give at least some advantages to those who adopt them. Should not special foods, vitamins, and other dietary supplements be banned along with steroids? No one protests that an athlete who regularly consumes junk food is being unfairly taken advantage of by his or her health-conscious competitor.

Drugs can harm health

According to Fost, one argument used by those who oppose the use of drugs in sports is that drugs are harmful to the health of athletes. The basis of this argument seems to be that anything that hurts an athlete should not be allowed. But, insists Fost, this is not a good argument. Most sports involve a certain amount of risk of injury. Some sports involve a moderate or high amount of risk. For instance, athletes who compete in contact sports like wrestling, football, and hockey often suffer serious or permanent injuries. Therefore, just participating in these sports can be dangerous to an athlete's health. Yet few people argue that these sports should not be played. For some athletes, the risk of competing is greater than the risk of taking certain

A woman participates in a tennis match. Many athletes seek to improve their performance through proper diet, vitamins and minerals, dedication, and training.

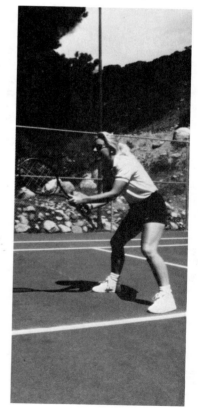

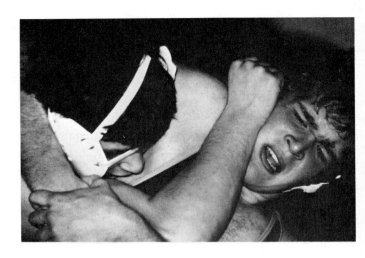

Two high school wrestlers vie for the championship during a Junior Varsity match. Studies suggest that the majority of high school students who use steroids hope to improve athletic performance. However, many athletes, such as these wrestlers, can improve their performance without the use of steroids.

drugs. Fost says that if a person is free to take part in dangerous sports, he or she should be just as free to take dangerous performance-enhancing drugs.

The fourteen-man football squad

Thomas H. Murray of the University of Texas disagrees with Fost. Murray contends that the ban on steroids should continue. He believes that not only is it unsafe for athletes to use steroids, but it is also unfair to the athletes who do not want to use them.

According to Murray, one reason athletes take performance-enhancing drugs is that they feel they are forced to do so. Other athletes may be taking these drugs and perhaps running a sprint a fraction of a second faster. Murray says the athletes who do not want to use the drugs have two choices: They can stay away from drugs, in which case their chances of winning are slim. Or they can give in and take the drugs and remain on an equal footing with their opponents. Murray states that people can argue that they should have the freedom to do whatever they want with their own bodies, but the athlete who is forced to take drugs in order to win has had his or her freedom to be drug-free revoked. In addi-

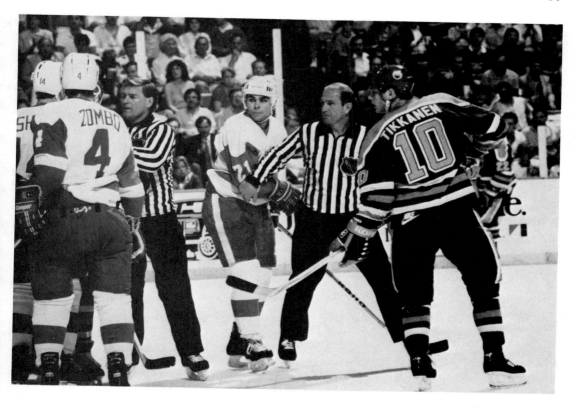

Spectators watch a hockey game. Although these players do not use steroids, some hockey players believe that steroids are a way of maintaining a competitive edge over opponents.

tion, Murray insists, once the drugs have taken their toll, these athletes have also lost the freedom to lead wholesome, happy lives.

Murray admits the existence of natural differences among athletes. But, he says, some ways of gaining an advantage over an opponent are obviously unnatural and unfair. For instance, it would be unfair for one shot-putter to use an eight-pound ball while his or her opponents use twelve-pounders. Similarly, it would be unfair for one football team to field fourteen players while the opposing team fields the usual eleven-player squad. In the same way, it is unfair for one person to benefit from a performance-enhancing drug while an opponent competes without it.

The arguments for and against steroid use continue both inside and outside the sports world.

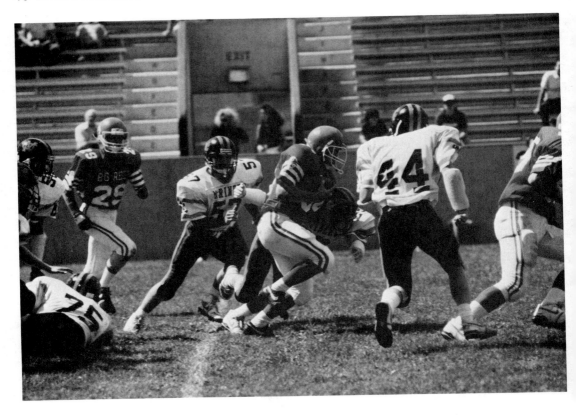

High school football players in action. These athletes advocate extensive training and a drug-free lifestyle as a means of improving athletic performance. Some football players, however, resort to steroid use to increase speed and strength and to heal injuries.

However, most medical doctors, coaches, and even athletes agree that steroid use can be dangerous. To combat this danger, federal and local government officials, as well as large athletic organizations, are beginning to crack down on illegal steroid use. The U.S. government launched a major attack on illegal steroids in 1985. More than twenty people have been convicted of dealing the drug and steroids worth millions of dollars have been seized by federal officials.

States are also getting tough on steroid use. In 1987, California officially classified steroids as controlled substances, a term used to designate dangerous drugs. Penalties were stiffened for illegal distribution of steroids.

Besides penalties, experts agree that education is

also needed to help eliminate steroid abuse. Dr. Stuart Nightengale, associate commissioner for Health Affairs for the Food and Drug Administration (FDA), remarked, "Americans haven't realized how harmful steroids are. Kids and adults are using these drugs without knowing what they're all about." Responding to this knowledge gap, the FDA and the Department of Education have begun a program for public awareness about steroids. Posters and newsletters have been sent to almost every grade school and high school in the United States.

Some private gyms are not waiting to be forced into discouraging steroid use. Instead, these gyms have begun to regulate themselves. For example, at Chicago's B&W Gym, a sign reads: "There are a

High school soccer players compete for control of the ball. Although these players do not use steroids, medical experts believe that steroid use by young athletes is on the rise. Steroid use by adolescents is dangerous.

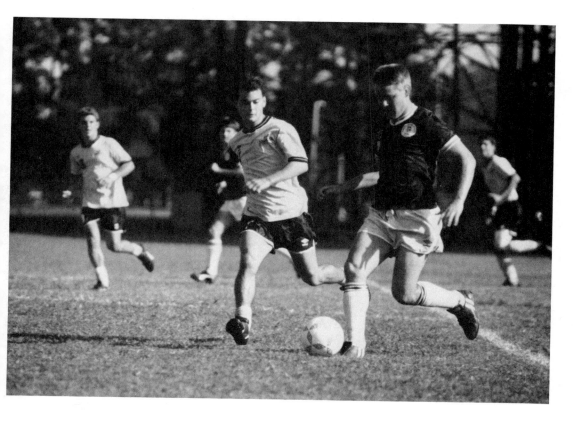

Dennis Banks teaches a physical education class at the Loneman School in South Dakota. Banks believes that it is important to discourage steroid use in young children.

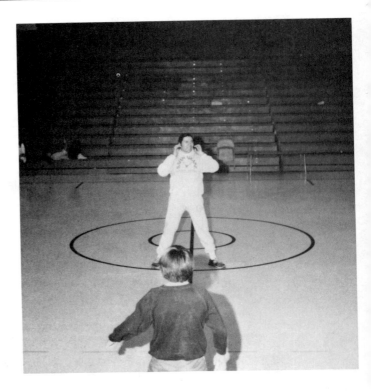

lot of gyms in Chicago that think steroids are okay. This isn't one of them." Dennis Brady, owner of the gym, says, "It's not fair. A fellow who's trained hard for years gets obliterated by a guy who's been lifting a year and taking 'juice.'"

The future of steroids

It is difficult to tell how prevalent steroids will become in the future. Perhaps they will become so widespread that most people will just accept or at least tolerate them. This is what happened with nicotine in cigarettes and caffeine in coffee and colas. That would please Dan Duchaine, who says, "I would like to make steroid use an old term and steroid therapy an accepted term."

Or perhaps public outrage will increase until steroids are effectively banned and their use subsides. That would have pleased the late Dr. John

Ziegler, one of the first people to introduce steroids to athletes in the United States. That was before the adverse health effects of steroids became known. Ziegler later regretted advising young athletes to take steroids. Before his death in 1983, Ziegler commented, "I wish I had never heard the word 'steroid.' These kids don't realize the terrible price they are going to pay."

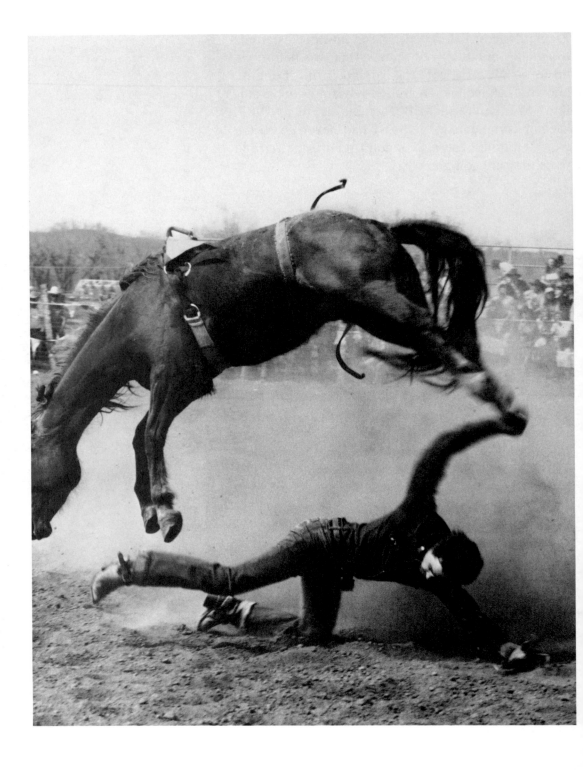

4

Playing Hard and Partying Even Harder: Alcohol in Sports

CHRIS MULLIN had been a star basketball player at St. John's University in Jamaica, New York. He had won the college basketball Player of the Year Award. Mullin did all the things an athlete was supposed to do. He practiced hard and played hard. He also drank hard. "Where I come from in Brooklyn," Mullin says, "beer was like water. You drank it at weddings, and you drank it at funerals. You drank 'cause you were happy, or 'cause you were sad." Former baseball pitcher Bob Lemon had made the same point when he said, "You drank after wins, you drank after losses, and you drank after rain-outs."

Sportswriter Mike Lupica agrees. "The fact is," he says, "sports are built for drinking. The sporting life and the drinking life have always gone together like Scotch and soda. The notion that you can play hard and then party even harder is . . . a part of the romance of sports." Chris Mullin continued to be one of the boys. He persisted in drinking to excess.

A bucking horse throws its rider during a rodeo in Montana. After a sporting event such as this, some athletes drink alcohol to relax and to deaden the pain of aching muscles.

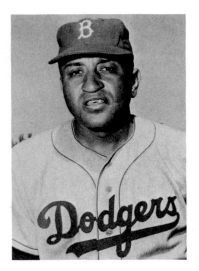

Pitcher Don Newcombe of the Brooklyn Dodgers poses in 1956. Newcombe believes that alcohol abuse is a problem among athletes, and that his own drinking problem shortened his career.

Then, in December of 1987, Mullin suddenly stopped drinking. "I finally figured something out," he said. "I wasn't one of the boys. I was an alcoholic."

Because alcohol is legal and its use accepted in society, many people tend to forget that it is a drug. Don Newcombe, who says his major league baseball career was cut short by alcohol use, states, "Everybody wants to do something about the drug problem in sports, but they just sort of wink at the main drug, which is alcohol."

Other athletes have also suffered from alcohol use. In 1988, Los Angeles Rams player and former Heisman trophy winner Charles White was suspended for testing positive for alcohol. And in December 1989, Billy Martin, former manager of the New York Yankees, died in a traffic accident in New York state. He and the driver of the truck were drunk.

Alcohol abuse

Alcohol is classified as a depressant drug because it acts to depress, or slow, the functions of the brain and nervous system. In small, occasional doses, the drug has not been shown to be harmful to most people. But consumed in larger amounts and more frequently, alcohol has caused problems because it is both physically and psychologically addictive. Over the years, many heavy drinkers have suffered the physical, emotional, and social ravages of alcoholism—dependency on alcohol. Recovery for alcoholics is usually a long and difficult process.

Alcohol is the most abused drug in the United States. It has been estimated that more than thirteen million Americans have serious alcohol problems. Under the influence of the drug, normal reaction time can become impaired. This leads to a high accident rate for those who become intoxicated. Half of all traffic fatalities and one-third of all traffic injuries are related to alcohol use.

Unlike steroids and other performance-enhancing drugs like caffeine, alcohol does not make athletes perform better. Some players feel the drug relaxes them. But most athletes learn quickly that any benefits that might come from feeling relaxed are offset by the reduced muscle coordination caused by drinking alcohol. Clearly then, athletes do not drink to play better.

Why do athletes drink?

Perhaps one reason athletes drink is because advertisers often promote the image that alcohol and sports go together. For instance, beer companies sponsor many sports events. Their advertisements show popular, professional athletes enjoying themselves with a beer. These ads tell the general public that drinking is acceptable and harmless because clean-cut, healthy athletes drink. But it also tells athletes that drinking is a requirement in athletics. The message to athletes is that if they want to be popular sports figures, they should drink alcohol.

Another reason athletes drink is peer pressure. Like Chris Mullin, many want to "fit in" with friends or teammates. If their friends or teammates are drinking alcohol, they feel they have to drink too. They want to be one of the crowd. Baseball player Dennis Martinez says, "I was one of the boys until I got arrested."

Martinez was arrested for driving while intoxicated in 1983. Alcohol had almost ruined his career. Luckily, he quit drinking and made a comeback. "If I hadn't stopped drinking," says Martinez, "I'd be out of baseball. I'd have lost my family, my job; I'd be on the street dying like everybody else." Martinez believes that a major reason so many baseball players drink is that they do not realize the harm it can cause. "Nobody in baseball wants to be-

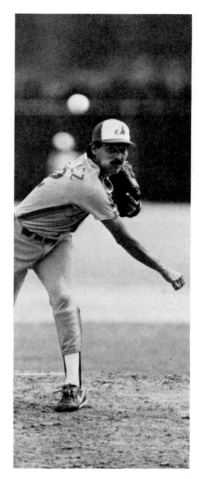

Baseball player Dennis Martinez throws a pitch during the 1989 season. In 1983, Martinez was arrested for driving under the influence of alcohol.

lieve how dangerous alcohol is. They say, 'I'm okay, I drink, I don't do drugs.' They don't realize that alcohol is the number one killer in the world."

No athlete knows better how dangerous alcohol can be than former world-class diver Bruce Kimball. Kimball came from a family of divers and began training at the age of two. By the time he was thirteen, he placed fourteenth at the Olympic trials. Then, in 1981, while he was a freshman in college, his car was struck head-on by a drunk driver. All the bones in Kimball's face shattered, his spleen ruptured, and his left leg fractured. His family, friends, and doctors thought he would never dive again. But Kimball was not ready to quit. He endured months of painful surgery and physical therapy, then began diving every day. In an amazing comeback, he won the silver medal at the 1984 Olympics. The experts said he had a chance for the gold in Seoul in 1988.

The wrecked car of world-class diver Bruce Kimball. In 1988, while intoxicated, Kimball killed two people when he drove his car into a group of pedestrians.

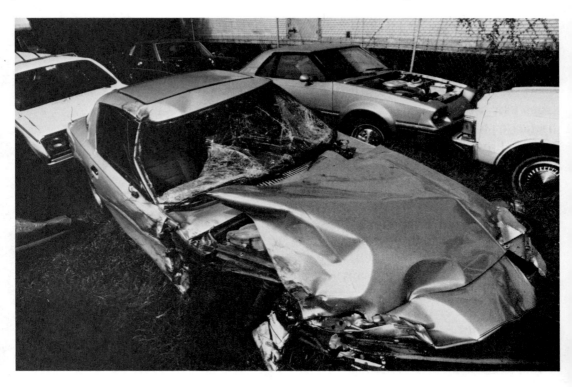

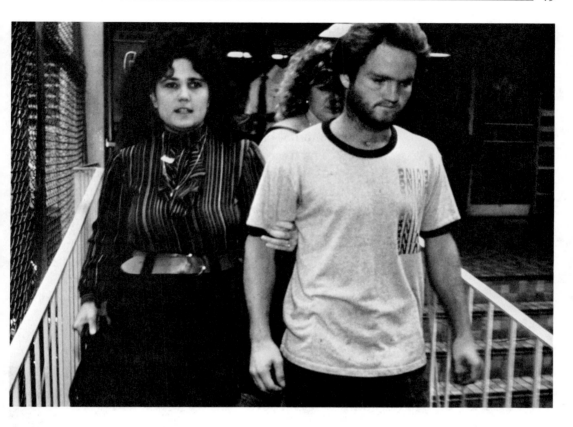

But Kimball apparently did not learn from his misfortune. On August 1, 1988, while intoxicated, he drove his car at a speed of nearly ninety miles per hour in a thirty-five-mile-per-hour zone. Losing control, he smashed into a group of young people, killing two and seriously injuring six others. For one young athlete, alcohol brought an abrupt end to a promising career.

The career of Bruce Kimball came to an abrupt end when he was forced to serve prison time after his drunk-driving accident.

Physical effects of alcohol

As is true with the general population, athletes who drink can sometimes drink too much. They are then at risk of developing the physical conditions that result from repeated alcohol use.

Drinking alcohol does not affect everyone in exactly the same way. Some people can "hold their liquor" better than other people. However, doctors agree that excessive use of the drug will eventually lead to serious complications.

Alcohol can injure the stomach lining, causing vomiting and bleeding. Stomach and intestinal ulcers (sores) often afflict heavy drinkers and can lead to internal bleeding.

The liver is directly damaged by repeated alcohol consumption. If the drinking stops, the liver can repair some or all of the damage. But if the person continues to use the drug, cirrhosis of the liver can develop. Cirrhosis is a severe scarring of liver tissue. In advanced cases, the liver can no longer function properly. The result is weakness, fluid buildup in the abdomen, and coma. Because the liver is essential to life, cirrhosis can eventually lead to death.

Alcohol also harms the brain and nerves. Tests have shown that excessive use of the drug destroys

Alcohol abuse is a serious problem in our society. Some people become dependent on alcohol, both physically and psychologically.

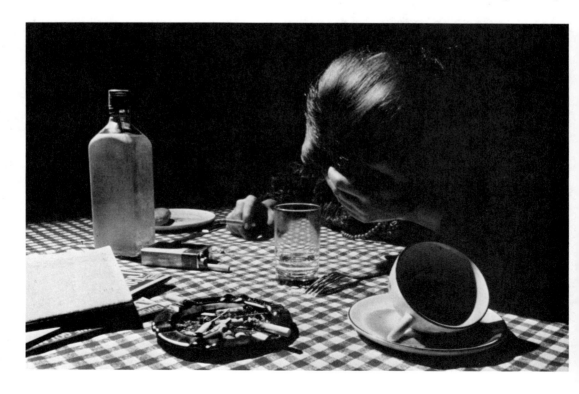

brain cells that control coordination and reflexes. This is especially damaging to athletes, who rely on these capabilities to compete. Nerves in the arms and legs can also suffer damage. This causes pain in the hands and feet. Severe abuse of alcohol can also result in a decrease in the ability to reason clearly.

In addition, alcohol can cause weakening of muscle tissue, especially in large muscles like those in the thigh. In serious cases, walking can become difficult. Since the heart is a muscle, it too can become weakened. Heart failure can occur, particularly if an unusually large amount of alcohol is consumed at one time.

Alcohol and malnutrition

Another problem encountered by people who use alcohol regularly is malnutrition. People who drink a lot of alcohol tend to eat less than they should. They may be consuming plenty of calories each day, but it is alcohol, not food, that is supplying these calories. Since alcoholic beverages contain few essential nutrients, such as proteins, vitamins, and minerals, people who drink alcohol and do not eat properly can become malnourished. Lack of proper nourishment can be especially harmful to athletes. Their bodies tend to need more nutrients than those of nonathletes because they are more active. A prolonged lack of nutrients can weaken an athlete's body so that competition becomes impossible.

Most of the complications mentioned thus far occur as a result of frequent alcohol use. But even short-term use can have a negative effect on an athlete's performance. Drinking alcohol before a game or competition can impair an athlete's psychomotor abilities. These include reaction time, hand-eye coordination, accuracy, balance, and motor skills. Sports most affected by reduction of these abilities

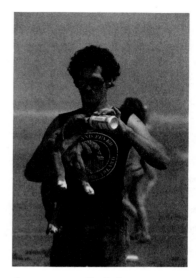

A young man feeds beer to a dog during spring break in Texas. Some people believe that young people are influenced by advertisements linking clean-cut athletes with beer.

are those that require quick reactions to changing situations. Basketball, hockey, football, tennis, and auto racing are examples.

Beating alcohol abuse

Some athletes have been forced out of their careers by alcohol and drugs. "From the beginning, I was out of control," says former major league baseball pitcher Sam McDowell. But he did not care. "The more you drank, the more you were a man, right? The harder you played on the field, the harder you played off it, that's what I thought." "Sudden" Sam McDowell managed to strike out 2,453 batters in 2,492 innings. All the while, he was an alcoholic and a drug addict. Then his addiction caught up with him. He had to quit major league baseball at the age of thirty-three, at the height of his career.

McDowell eventually got help for himself and learned to help others. He became an addiction counselor for athletes. He sees the elimination of alcohol and other drugs from sports as a long, difficult process. He believes that addiction counselors like himself should be on hand at training camps and locker rooms to support athletes who have alcohol problems. "I'm talking about education," he says, "and intervention when necessary." By intervention, McDowell means having counselors or teammates keep a close watch on players who need help.

But McDowell admits that the problem is widespread and deep-rooted. As long as the public and the beer companies continue to strengthen the connection between alcohol and athletics, players will become hooked. "We may be ten or twenty years of education away from getting a handle on this thing. There's big money in alcoholism. Look around you in sports," he said.

Chris Mullin put himself into a treatment center.

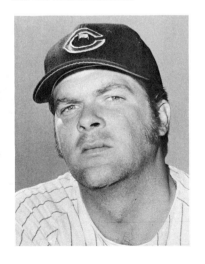

Pitcher Sam McDowell admits that he was an alcoholic and drug addict while he played for the Cleveland Indians.

Many other athletes have done the same. Some have managed to remain drug-free. Others have not. Mullin believes athletes can avoid alcohol dependency by being honest with themselves. "Sure, I put up these phony barriers for myself," says Mullin. "First, I wouldn't drink before a game. . . . I had these, you know, *Nevers*. Never on Sunday. Never the night before the game. But then, you start to get rid of them. . . you'd say, couple of beers tonight won't hurt me. Or two nights in a row won't hurt me. . . then, instead of two days in a row, it was three."

Mullin, McDowell, and dozens of other athletes who have admitted to being alcoholics, see education as the major way to fight alcohol abuse. The first step, they say, is getting society as a whole to recognize that alcohol is a dangerous drug. Perhaps then athletes will be more inclined to think about the risks they are taking when they drink.

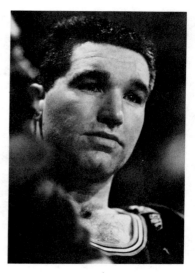

Chris Mullin, a basketball player at St. John's University, put himself into a treatment center after admitting to a drinking problem.

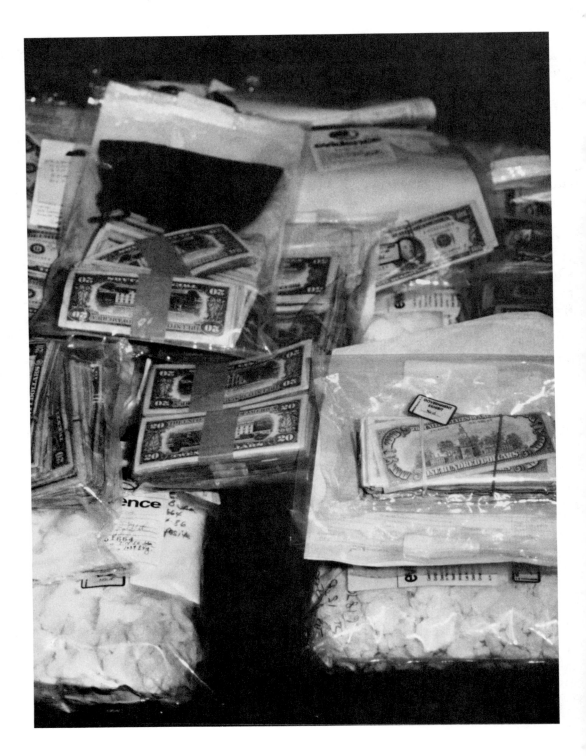

5

Cocaine: A Quick High Followed by a Long Nightmare

PERHAPS THE MOST widely publicized recreational drug is cocaine. The National Institute on Drug Abuse (NIDA) estimates that about six million Americans use cocaine regularly. These include people in every profession. But professional athletes who use the drug both for recreation and as an energy booster before games have been hit unusually hard by the drug. "Seemingly indestructible heroes have been brought to their knees," says William Gildea, a sportswriter for *The Washington Post*. Gildea describes the use of cocaine by some athletes as "a nightmare of physical suffering, depression and paranoia, craving cocaine more than life itself. . . . Once they had fame, fortune, secure futures. Now all that is left is shattered lives—and sometimes not even that."

Most successful athletes are young, strong, and popular. Some of them think nothing can hurt them, not even drugs. If a person offers them cocaine, they might figure it is all right to try it. But, warns Gildea, "Cocaine can creep up on you, and it won't let go. All it takes to get hooked is money and free time—two things professional athletes have a lot of."

Crack, shown here with some trafficking profits, is taken for its euphoriant effect. Medical experts believe that this form of cocaine is highly addictive.

55

Consider the case of Larry Bethea, a bright and talented football star from Newport News, Virginia. Bethea stood six feet five inches tall and weighed 220 pounds while still in high school. He was a favorite of teachers and a member of the National Honor Society. When he played for Michigan State, he was named the Big Ten Conference's most valuable player.

In 1978, Bethea was the number one draft choice of the Dallas Cowboys. He received a six-figure bonus and married his high school sweetheart. Then, when everything in his life seemed to be going well, he suddenly began using drugs.

By 1980, Bethea used cocaine often, and his life had begun to crumble. His coaches felt his playing was so uninspired that they benched him. He started freebasing cocaine, or smoking the drug directly through a pipe, rather than inhaling the powder. His

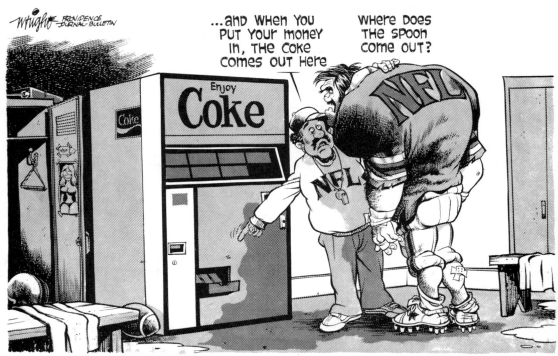

wife asked for a divorce.

In 1986, no longer able to play football, Bethea returned to Newport News and moved in with his mother. Not long afterward, he was arrested for stealing sixty-four thousand dollars from her. The judge gave him a suspended sentence.

On April 22, 1987, Bethea stole a .38-caliber handgun and held up two local convenience stores. Because the stores were in his own neighborhood, the clerks recognized him immediately. At 1:40 the next morning, police found Bethea in a pool of blood behind a run-down boardinghouse known to be a hangout for drug addicts. The hometown hero with a life and future most people only dream about had put the pistol to his head and pulled the trigger.

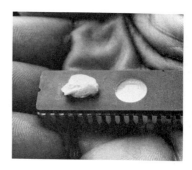

Crack, a very pure form of cocaine, rests on a measuring device in the palm of a man's hand. Crack produces a short, but intense, state of exhilaration.

Instant addiction

The rise and tragic fall of Larry Bethea may seem like an unusually horrifying case. But in today's world of cocaine addiction, such stories are becoming more and more common. Like Len Bias and Don Rogers, Bethea became one more terrible statistic in the growing battle between cocaine and society.

Like caffeine, cocaine is a stimulant. It can make a person feel awake and alert and produce a brief state of exhilaration, or pleasurable excitement. But these feelings are short-lived, as the effects of cocaine wear off rapidly. To maintain a cocaine "high," the user must repeatedly ingest the drug, and cocaine is highly addictive. Some people can become cocaine addicts after only a few days of repeated use. Others take longer to get hooked, but prolonged use causes addiction eventually.

Cocaine is extracted from the leaves of the coca plant, a small bush that commonly grows wild in the South American countries of Bolivia, Peru and Colombia. For hundreds of years, the Indians of the area chewed the leaves of the coca plant. Sometimes they did this for pleasure. Other reasons for taking the drug were to relieve the boredom of hard physical labor or to ward off hunger and thirst. The drug can deaden feeling in the stomach lining so that a person does not notice he or she is hungry.

In 1884, in Vienna, Austria, Carl Koller became the first person to use cocaine as a local anesthetic. He found that it effectively deadened nerves in the mucous membranes of the eye, nose, and throat. This medical use of cocaine spread quickly and became common in many countries. But recreational use of the drug also spread quickly. By the early years of the twentieth century, cocaine addiction had become a problem in many of the world's largest cities.

In the 1960s, there was a sharp increase in cocaine abuse and addiction in the United States and other developed countries. This was due to the introduction of more potent and, at the same time, cheaper versions of the drug.

Cocaine can be used in many forms

Cocaine abusers most often sniff, or "snort," a powdered form of the drug. They can also inject it after it has been dissolved in a solution. And the drug is also taken orally or freebased. An unusually pure form of cocaine called "crack" has become popular. When smoked in a pipe or mixed with tobacco in a cigarette, it makes a popping sound, which is why it was nicknamed crack. Because it is so pure, crack delivers an intense high lasting three to five minutes after being taken. This form of cocaine appears to be instantly addictive.

The most obvious and immediate effect of sniffing cocaine is damage to the nasal cavity, the inside of the nose. With repeated use of the drug, ulcerations, which are serious sores that do not heal well,

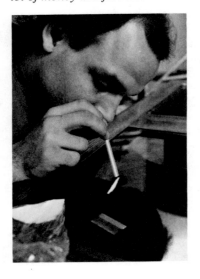

A young athlete snorts cocaine. Some people believe that athletes are especially prone to cocaine use because they have a lot of money and free time.

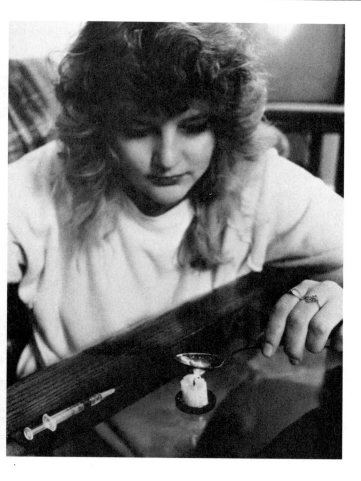

A woman dissolves cocaine over a candle. When in liquid form, the drug can be injected directly into the bloodstream.

can appear in the mucous membranes of the cavity. Pain and bleeding are common side effects.

Frequent cocaine users can experience episodes of shaking and sweating. They can become restless and easily angered. Another common problem of users is insomnia, the inability to fall asleep. Also, anxiety afflicts many people who abuse the drug.

As larger amounts of cocaine are taken in, the spinal cord itself can become stimulated. The user might then go into convulsions, in which whole sections of the body violently and repeatedly tighten and relax. Sometimes the entire nervous system can be so affected by the drug that normal breathing becomes impossible. In such cases, death can quickly follow.

Because cocaine can cause someone to feel worried, even fearful, most users feel more comfortable taking the drug in the company of other people. Addicts often persuade friends to join in. This creates peer pressure some individuals cannot resist. Many nonusers give in and try the drug just to satisfy their user friends. Soon, the nonusers have become users too. This is one common way such drug abuse spreads through society.

Cocaine use can be especially risky for athletes because it can impair judgment. Sports competitors need to be able to accurately judge distance, height, and time duration. For instance, a soccer player must be able to calculate mentally when, where, and how the ball will move in order to hit it with his head. Drug-induced judgment problems can sometimes be dangerous to the athlete as well as to his or her opponents and fans. For example, a race car driver who has taken drugs before a race risks losing control of the car and crashing. The driver, his or her competitors, and even spectators can be injured or killed.

The personal impact of cocaine

Athletes often do not realize they are hooked on cocaine until they have lost their careers and families. Former Denver Nuggets basketball star David Thompson thought he was immune to drug addiction. "You never feel like you're going to be the one to get hooked," Thompson said. But the man who had once been the highest paid player in the National Basketball Association (NBA) at $800,000 a season *did* get hooked on cocaine. Thompson explains, "Your use becomes greater and greater. It really affected the way I played. Sometimes I wasn't so much into the game as into what was going to

Soccer players compete for the ball. These players abstain from drug use, because they know it is detrimental to athletes who must be able to judge distance and other factors.

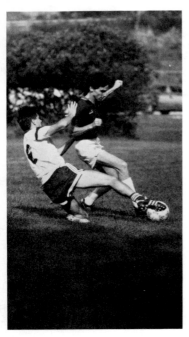

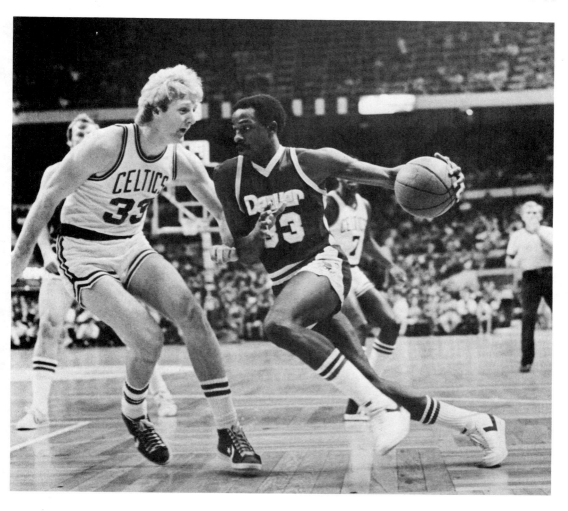

happen after the game. I knew it was harmful both for me and for my career, but I couldn't stop."

Thompson not only lost his career, but also his family life. The drug affected his relationships with his parents, wife, and daughters. He was arrested for assault, spent months in jail, and had to file for bankruptcy, listing more than $2 million in debts. Most of the money had been spent on drugs. After getting out of jail, Thompson was asked what he would say to someone thinking about trying cocaine. The answer: "Never try it. It's easy to get in-

David Thompson of the Denver Nuggets drives hard past Boston Celtics' Larry Bird during a game at the Boston Garden. Thompson lost his career after getting hooked on cocaine.

volved with, and it's very hard to get out of."

One athlete who could not get out of the grip of cocaine is Washington Redskins defensive end Dexter Manley. In 1989, he tested positive for cocaine. This was the third time he had violated the NFL's substance abuse policy. The previous violations had occurred in 1987 and 1988. In accordance

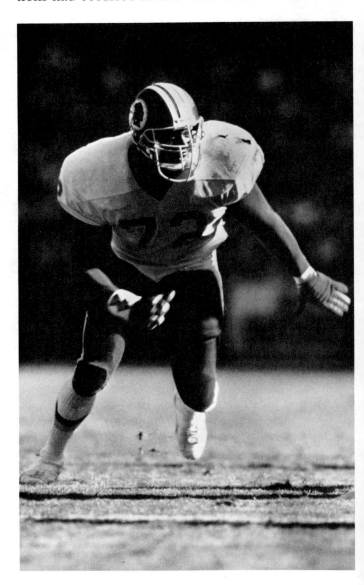

In 1989, Washington Redskins defensive end Dexter Manley was suspended from professional football after testing positive for cocaine.

with the league's rules, Manley was suspended from professional football.

Other athletes have paid a high price for cocaine use. In 1979, Dallas Cowboy star Bob Hayes was convicted on two counts of selling cocaine. In 1983, Eugene "Mercury" Morris of the Miami Dolphins was sentenced to twenty years for the same charge. In 1983-1984, Willie Aikens, Jerry Martin, and Willie Wilson of the Kansas City Royals each served 81-day sentences for attempting to buy cocaine.

One of the lucky ones

A handful of athletes has managed to recover from devastating cocaine-related problems. One is former football great Carl Eller, who has been described as one of the greatest defensive ends ever to play the game. At six feet six inches and 255 pounds, he helped the Minnesota Vikings reach the Super Bowl four times between 1969 and 1976. One teammate called Eller's playing "unbelievable."

Intelligent and hard-working, Eller invested much of his money in real estate. Eventually, his net worth was estimated at $3 million. But, by the mid-1970s, Eller had begun to invest his money in cocaine. "The glamour and good times got to Eller; he began to think of himself the same way others saw him, as simply indestructible," according to sportswriter William Gildea.

By 1977, Eller was freebasing cocaine. His habit now cost him two thousand dollars a week, and his playing suffered. His business and real estate deals began to fall apart. Cocaine finally caused him to lose weight and upper-body strength, and he had to quit football. Like David Thompson, Eller declared bankruptcy. Eventually, Eller was persuaded to enter a drug-treatment center. But even though the co-

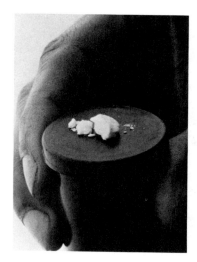

Cocaine, shown here in the hand of an athlete, can make a user feel awake and alert.

Former football player Carl Eller declared bankruptcy after spending thousands of dollars on his cocaine habit.

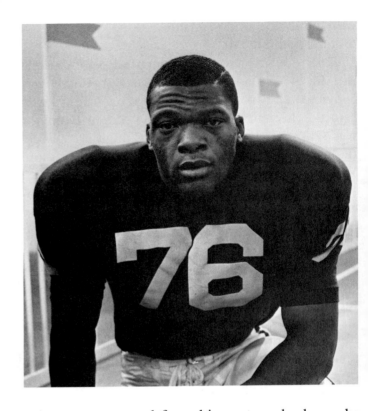

caine was removed from his system, he knew he was not cured. He realized he would have to fight the craving for the drug each day for the rest of his life. But Eller realized something else, something many professional athletes never discover. He learned that Carl Eller the human being was worth just as much as Carl Eller the football star. He decided to help other players find their own self-worth.

At the suggestion of former NFL commissioner Pete Rozelle, Eller lectured the NFL team owners at one of their annual meetings. He shocked them with his stories of cocaine abuse by players on every team. Eller began talking to teams and players, trying to convince those using cocaine to stop and others not to start. Finally, he opened his own drug-rehabilitation center in the Minneapolis-St. Paul area.

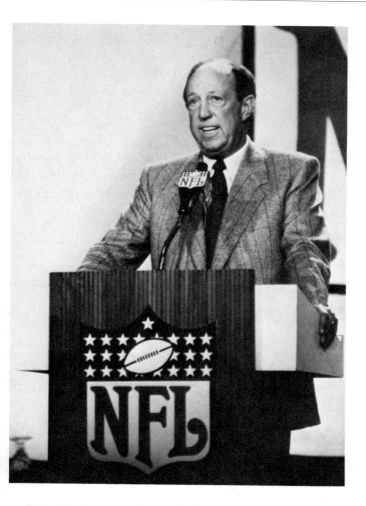

Pete Rozelle, former NFL commissioner, talks to NFL owners. Rozelle encouraged Carl Eller to tell others about the negative effects of cocaine.

Eller believes reformed drug users like himself can have an impact on the problem of drugs in sports. They can tell potential drug users where the rocky road of drug abuse can lead because they have been down that road. Eller tells athletes what cocaine can do to their lives. "There's no comparison between the amount of money I make now and what I once made," he says. "But I'm one of the lucky ones. I could have ended up in jail—or dead."

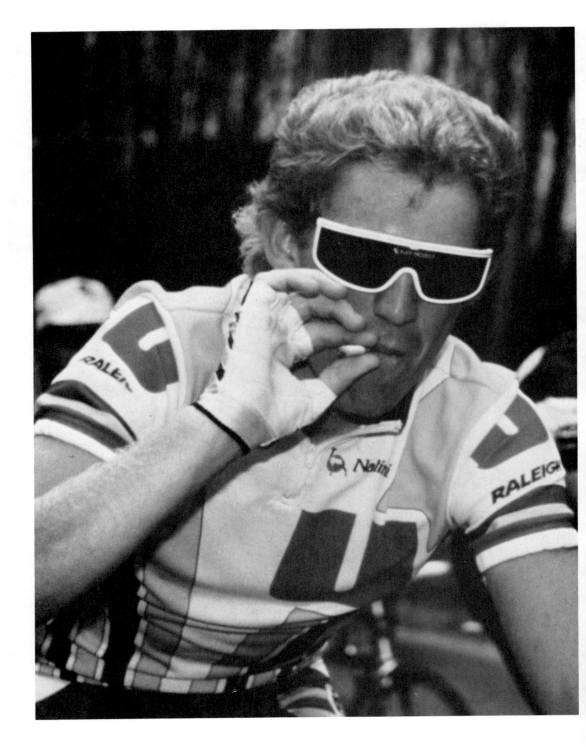

6

Drugs That Tend to Be Ignored

STEROIDS, COCAINE, and alcohol are the drugs that seem to get most of the attention in the media. Perhaps that is because these drugs so often wreck the lives of famous people. Also, for various reasons, the focus of attention on specific drugs changes from decade to decade. For instance, in the 1960s, marijuana was a highly publicized and debated drug. During the 1980s, the media and drug officials shifted attention to drugs like cocaine, which was perceived as more widespread and harmful. This can be deceiving, for the use of less publicized drugs is not necessarily less common or less dangerous.

Nicotine

Consider nicotine, which is one of the most widely consumed legal drugs. Nicotine is found in tobacco products, including cigarettes, cigars, chewing (smokeless) tobacco, and snuff, a powdered form of tobacco that is sniffed. A poisonous chemical, nicotine is highly addictive, often causing dependence after only a few weeks of use.

The most common form of tobacco use, cigarette smoking, is the leading cause of preventable illness in the developed countries. Smoking leads to cancer, heart disease, and emphysema and is account-

A cyclist puffs on a cigarette during the Tour de France in 1989.

able for more than one thousand deaths per day in the United States alone. Statistics show that cigarettes constitute a far more serious health threat than cocaine or other illegal drugs. For instance, in 1985, there were 300,000 tobacco-related deaths in the United States, as compared to 643 reported cocaine-related deaths. Yet, like alcohol, tobacco is legal and socially acceptable. Thus, for many young people, including some young athletes, experimenting with tobacco seems a perfectly natural thing to do.

Tobacco use by athletes

Athletes learned early about smoking tobacco. They found that it causes shortness of breath and lowers stamina. For instance, runners who smoke cannot run as far as nonsmoking runners. The smokers also get tired sooner. For these reasons, few professional or collegiate athletes smoke. However, the problem persists on the high school and junior high school levels. High school coach Steve Goveia estimates that "about 5 to 10 percent of high school athletes smoke, although there seems to be a recent, noticeable decline in smoking by boys. On the other hand, smoking among school-age female athletes and cheerleaders has increased dramatically."

Athletes also engage in chewing smokeless tobacco. Baseball players and wrestlers have traditionally been heavy users of the substance. The sight of a baseball pitcher spitting tobacco juice on the mound has become a familiar image in popular culture. "It is hard to imagine watching a baseball game without references to chewing tobacco. During one of the 1986 World Series games, there were almost twenty-four minutes of air time devoted to players and coaches chewing and dipping smokeless tobacco," said sports doctor Gary Green.

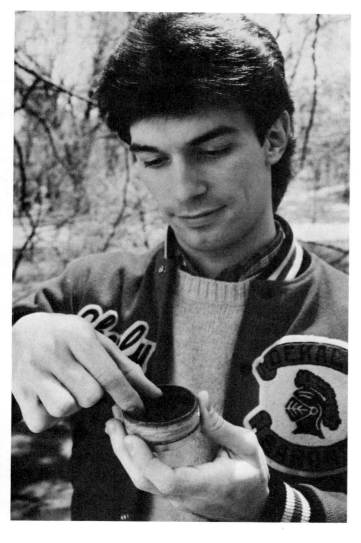

A young athlete pinches chewing tobacco from a tin. Many people believe that this form of tobacco is not addictive, even though it contains as much nicotine as cigarettes.

In recent years, the use of chewing tobacco by young athletes has increased, mainly because of the influence of professional players who use the product. Another reason for its popularity is the common myth that chewing is relatively safe when compared to smoking. Younger athletes in particular seem to think they will not become addicted to chewing tobacco. But the substance contains as much nicotine as any other form of tobacco and causes addiction

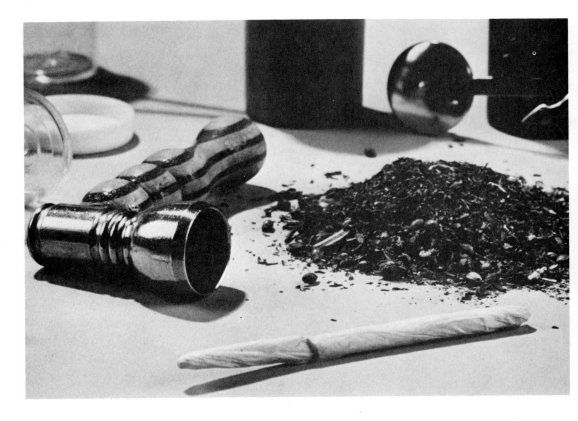

Marijuana is an illegal drug that is usually smoked in cigarettes or pipes. It can also be sniffed or eaten. It is used for its intoxicating effect, but even low doses can impair short-term memory, perception, and behavior.

in a majority of regular users. Also, studies have shown that users of smokeless tobacco have rates of mouth cancer fifty times higher than normal. At least one young athlete died as a result of cancer of the mouth caused by chewing tobacco.

Chewing tobacco and cancer

Sean Marsee, a high school senior from Ada, Oklahoma, had won many medals as a star runner on the school track team. He had also chewed tobacco since the age of thirteen. In 1983, Sean's doctor examined a large sore in his mouth and ordered tests done. The diagnosis was oral cancer. Sean underwent three operations. But the cancer had already spread into too many areas of his body. He died on February 25, 1984. Sean had become one of the nine thousand Americans who die each year from oral cancer. Health officials suspect that many of these deaths may be due to the use of smokeless tobacco.

Keep off the grass

Marijuana, a drug that was especially popular during the 1960s and 1970s, is also used by athletes. Because marijuana is illegal, its detection in an athlete's system can mean not only suspension from his or her team but also a jail sentence. But that has not stopped many athletes from using it. Lance Rentzel of the Los Angeles Rams, Calvin Thomas of the Chicago Bears, and Kevin Gogan of the Dallas Cowboys were suspended from their teams for pos-

Lung tissue samples from a non-smoker (left) and a smoker (right) indicate the detrimental effects of tobacco. The air sacs, which absorb oxygen, are not visible in normal lung tissue. Lung tissue of a smoker shows greatly enlarged air sacs, indicating damage to the lung.

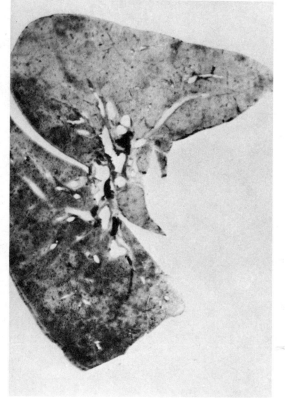
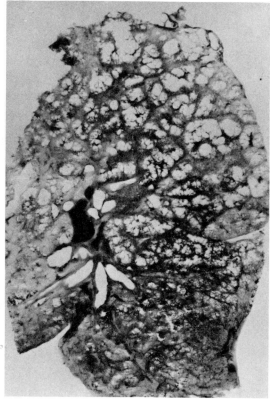

sessing and using marijuana. Orlando Cepeda, former first baseman with the San Francisco Giants and the St. Louis Cardinals, suffered more than suspension. In 1978, Cepeda was arrested and charged with importing and possessing marijuana. He served nine months in jail.

Marijuana is derived from the hemp plant, which grows on most continents, including Asia; Europe; and North, Central, and South America. It is usually smoked, either in cigarette papers or through a pipe. Hashish, or "hash," is a more powerful pastelike form of the drug and is also smoked. Commonly called "grass" or "pot," marijuana is classified as a hallucinogen. This is because after taking large

Cigarette consumption continues despite its health hazards. Although nicotine is a stimulant, many young people claim that smoking relaxes them.

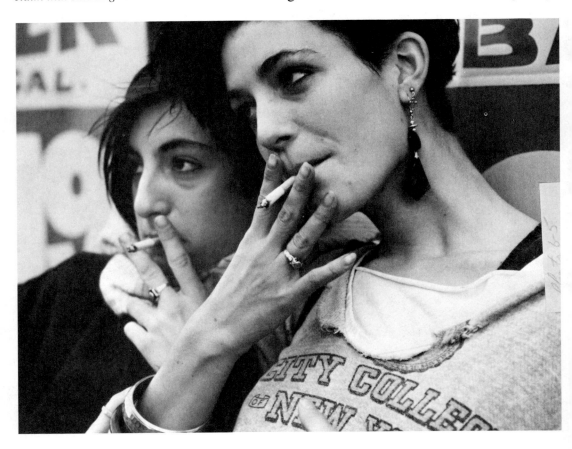

doses some users experience hallucinations. These are unpredictable changes in the way users see and hear things. Using smaller doses, most people report temporary feelings of well-being, followed by drowsiness. A few marijuana users become afraid. Some people who use the drug regularly for long periods of time have been known to suffer from depression. Although it has not been shown that marijuana is physically addictive, it may be psychologically addictive. That is, some users believe they need to smoke it in order to cope with life.

Marijuana has physical as well as psychological effects on the body. It increases blood pressure, dilates the pupils of the eyes, and quickens the heartbeat. Smoking marijuana can also damage the lungs the same way smoking cigarettes does. Regular marijuana users are at high risk of developing bronchitis, emphysema, and lung cancer.

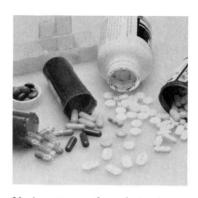

Various types of amphetamines, such as these, are used by some athletes to counteract fatigue and speed up performances.

Amphetamines

Another group of drugs used by athletes is amphetamines. Amphetamines are derived from the Ephedra plant, which grows mainly in desert regions. They are classified as stimulants, and because they can put people in an "up" mood, they are often called "uppers."

Amphetamines, although legal, are dangerous drugs and require a doctor's prescription. They are usually prescribed for people whose occupations demand that they remain awake and alert. For example, soldiers in battle have been given amphetamines to keep them from sleeping during times of danger. Because of their ability to deaden hunger, amphetamines have also been prescribed for weight loss.

Amphetamines affect the body much the way other stimulants do. That is, they cause the heart to beat faster and blood pressure to rise. This makes

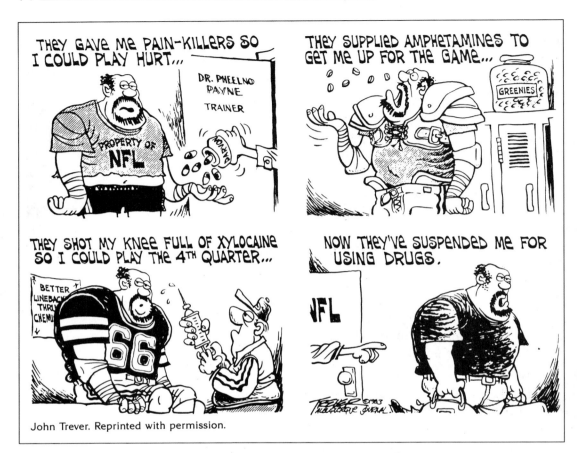

John Trever. Reprinted with permission.

the user feel energetic. Overuse of amphetamines can lead to addiction, mental illness, and even death.

Because of the energizing effects of amphetamines, some athletes use them while training and during competition. Amphetamine use has been tragic for at least two athletes. English cyclist Tommy Simpson and French cyclist Yves Mattin both died after consuming large amounts of amphetamines. Although many people believe amphetamine use by athletes has decreased in recent years, NBC sportscaster Tony Kubek says that the use of amphetamines among players "has never been higher."

A few athletes have also been affected by a little-publicized group of substances called "brake drugs." These are used in a drug treatment called "braking" that attempts to halt an athlete's growth. Thus, brake drugs have the opposite effect of steroids, which are used to stimulate growth. Reportedly, brake drugs have been used on young female gymnasts, especially in communist countries. These drugs appear to delay the onset of puberty, which causes young people's bodies to assume their adult proportions. The gymnasts taking the drugs tend to remain slender and petite well into their teen years. This supposedly gives them an advantage in gymnastic events that emphasize grace and agility. Other than delaying the onset of puberty, little is known about the effects brake drugs have on the body.

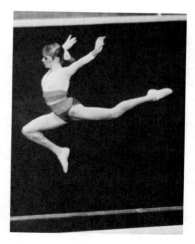

Gymnast Julianne McNamara leaps above a balancing beam. Some young gymnasts, although not McNamara, use drugs to halt their growth. These types of drugs, called brake drugs, delay puberty and allow the gymnast to remain agile and petite.

Media attention

Coaches and health officials alike believe the use of chewing tobacco, marijuana, amphetamines, and brake drugs all pose a serious problem in the sports world. Perhaps the media need to focus more attention on these less-publicized drugs. It is possible that when the general public as well as athletes become educated about the damage these drugs can do, they will take action to prevent their use.

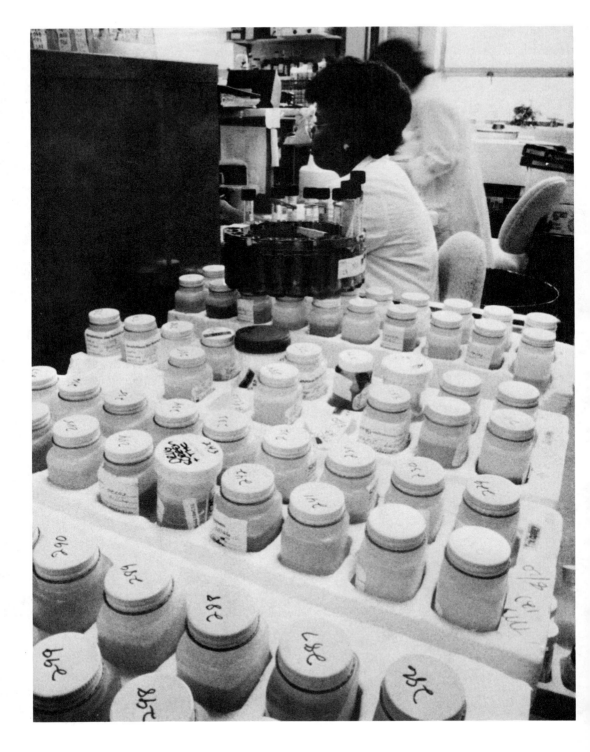

7

Drug Tests for Athletes: A Mounting Controversy

IN RECENT YEARS, many sports teams and organizations, recognizing the dangers of drug use, have instituted drug testing of athletes. In these tests, samples of urine or blood are examined for traces of various drugs. Those players who test positive often face suspensions, fines, and public humiliation.

There are arguments for and against drug testing. When a well-known sports figure is tested and found to have taken drugs, people tend to take sides. Some feel testing is a good thing and believe drug-using athletes should be punished. Others, including former NFL commissioner Pete Rozelle, think drug testing is not always accurate and can result in a wrong accusation and a damaged reputation. They also feel that such testing is an invasion of an athlete's privacy.

Ben Johnson's disqualification and loss of medals at the 1988 Seoul Olympics was one of the most publicized and debated incidents of drug testing. Officials of the International Olympic Committee

Urine samples are tested for the presence of drugs by technicians at the SmithKline Bio-Science Laboratories in Pennsylvania.

(IOC) and the International Amateur Athletic Federation (IAAF) stood by the test results and punished Johnson harshly. They took action against what they considered to be behavior unbecoming an athlete, especially one of Johnson's world-class stature.

Johnson's punishment is controversial

The officials were not alone. Many others approved of the testing and disciplining of Johnson. However, many also disagreed. They insisted that drug tests in sports are often inaccurate and therefore unfair. They pointed out that although other runners in Johnson's race had tested negative for steroids, there was still a possibility these runners had taken the drug. For instance, they could have stopped using steroids well before the tests, in time for the drugs to leave their systems. Maybe Johnson had just waited too long and traces of the drug remained in his system at the time of the test. Thus, say the antitest people, testing is often inconclusive and singles out for punishment those who are unable to beat the system.

Those against drug testing call attention to Johnson's 100-meter world record from 1987. At the time, he ran the race in 9.83 seconds at the World Championships in Rome. Recently, Johnson admitted to having taken steroids on many occasions since 1981, including one month before the 1987 race. Yet, after the race, he had tested negative for the drug, proving that athletes can outwit drug tests.

The antitest people also bring up another questionable drug test at the Seoul Olympics. Belgian marathoner Ria van Landeghem was accused of taking the steroid nandrolone. Apparently stunned by the charge, the runner demanded a second test. The results: negative for nandrolone but positive for an-

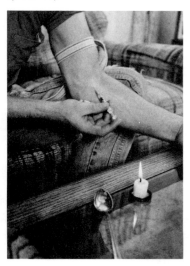

A young male injects cocaine. Some people believe drug testing will discourage this type of activity.

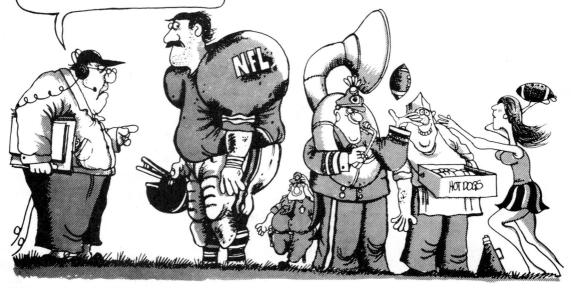

Ed Gamble. Reprinted with permission.

other type of steroid. Van Landeghem protested that she had never taken the drugs. But she was not allowed to compete and was given only two hours to pack her things and leave the Olympic Village.

Critics of the test insist it is strange to find single traces of two separate drugs during a two-day period. They suggest that van Landeghem's urine sample could have been mixed up with a sample belonging to another athlete. Van Landeghem herself contends that Belgian officials purposely fixed the tests so she would register positive. She claims they were angry with her for living and racing in the United States. Her case illustrates how a positive drug test, accurate or not, can affect an athlete's life and reputation.

Dr. Robert Voy, former chief medical officer for the U.S. Olympic Committee, thinks drug testing is necessary in athletics. He says testing for performance-enhancing drugs helps keep competition fair. Voy thinks athletes who use drugs like steroids have an unfair advantage over their opponents who do not use them. Testing allows officials to eliminate from competition those who have taken drugs, giving drug-free players a reasonable chance of winning.

Benefits of drug testing

Voy also believes drug testing may help preserve athletes' health and possibly even save their lives. Such testing might detect the presence of dangerous substances in their systems. Doctors could then administer treatment and educate the athletes as to the danger of the drugs they are using.

According to Voy, many young athletes will do almost anything to win. This sometimes includes destroying their own health. It is the responsibility of sports officials to try to keep this from happening. Voy uses the example of a weight lifter who trained to compete in the 1984 Olympics. The lifter took steroids to enhance his strength. While lifting, he dislocated his elbow, a common injury for lifters. Because he was thrown off balance, the barbell shifted and one of his legs had to support most of the weight. While steroids strengthen muscles, they do not strengthen tendons. A tendon in the lifter's lower leg ruptured, and he collapsed under the bar. The bar struck his head, injuring him seriously. Had he not taken steroids, he might not have attempted so heavy a lift and the tendon may have held.

Another pro-test argument centers around protecting athletes from poisonous substances. Many athletes travel all around the world and are exposed to types of drugs they have never heard of. For ex-

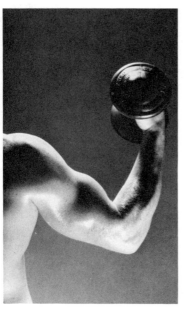

Advocates of drug testing believe that steroid use to build muscle mass is a dangerous practice.

ample, the drug strychnine is used in small doses as a stimulant in South America. While competing in a South American country, an athlete may be tempted to try this powerful substance. But he or she may not be aware that strychnine is highly poisonous in larger doses.

Similar to strychnine is caffeine, a stimulant taken by athletes as well as nonathletes to stay alert and boost energy levels. If taken in large enough doses, caffeine can be as deadly a poison as strychnine. Pro-test advocates say that a drug test that registers unusually high levels of strychnine or caffeine in a player's system can alert doctors to administer treatment. The player's health or life might be saved.

Drug testing saves lives

Dr. Allan Lans, a psychiatrist at St. Luke's-Roosevelt Hospital in New York City, agrees that testing athletes for drugs can help save their lives. "Testing should not be seen as a trap. It should be seen as a screen that's there to tell a player he's in trouble. It should be an aid," said Lans.

Jim Valvano, head basketball coach at North Carolina State University, also believes that athletes should be tested for drugs. "What surprises me," says Valvano, "is the amount of resistance to drug testing by people who say that it's a violation of individual freedoms. We're not talking about prayer in the school here, we're talking about life and death."

Another drug-testing advocate is Red Auerbach. About testing, Auerbach says, "I know that it's an invasion of privacy, but there comes a time when you've got to put this altruistic civil rights stuff down the toilet, find out who's using drugs and take it from there."

Jerry Tarkanian, head basketball coach at the

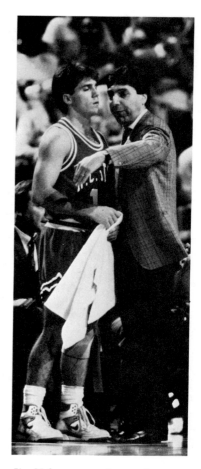

Jim Valvano coaches a player during a North Carolina State University game. Valvano advocates drug testing among athletes.

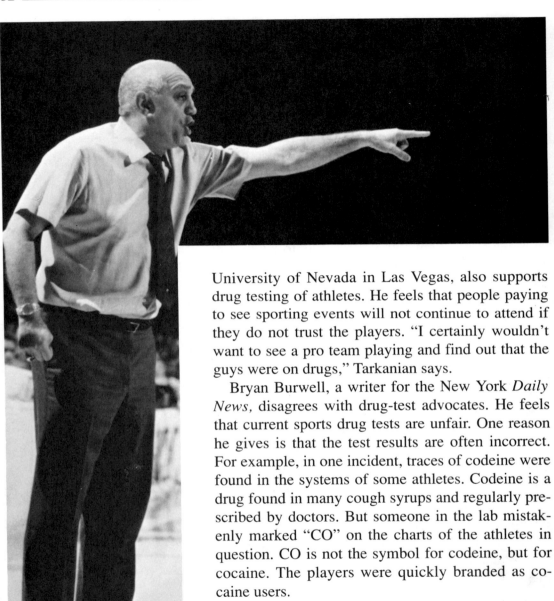

University of Nevada in Las Vegas, also supports drug testing of athletes. He feels that people paying to see sporting events will not continue to attend if they do not trust the players. "I certainly wouldn't want to see a pro team playing and find out that the guys were on drugs," Tarkanian says.

Bryan Burwell, a writer for the New York *Daily News,* disagrees with drug-test advocates. He feels that current sports drug tests are unfair. One reason he gives is that the test results are often incorrect. For example, in one incident, traces of codeine were found in the systems of some athletes. Codeine is a drug found in many cough syrups and regularly prescribed by doctors. But someone in the lab mistakenly marked "CO" on the charts of the athletes in question. CO is not the symbol for codeine, but for cocaine. The players were quickly branded as cocaine users.

Drug testing violates personal rights

Another reason Burwell is against drug testing involves the right to privacy. The results of drug tests are supposed to remain secret. However, athletes or managers sometimes start rumors about certain

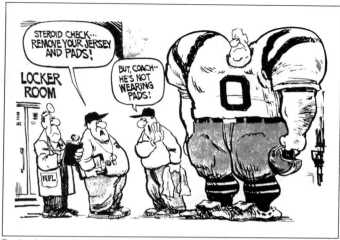

Reprinted with special permission of © 1989 North American Syndicate, Inc.

players testing positive. The players may or may *not* actually have tested positive, but when the names of these players reach the media, everyone assumes they *did* test positive. This is unfair to the athletes, who agreed to the tests after being assured the results would not reach the public.

Burwell tells the story of one athlete whose reputation was ruined, even though it was never proved he tested positive for drugs. Only two days after the announcement that James Fitzpatrick had been picked to play for the San Diego Chargers, a rumor spread that Fitzpatrick had tested positive for marijuana. The national news media picked up the story and people began assuming he was a drug addict.

When an athlete is accused of taking drugs, money as well as reputation can be lost. Alonzo Johnson, of the Philadelphia Eagles, is reported to have lost more than $500,000 in salary and bonuses after rumors spread that he was a drug user. Players can also lose money that they would have made by endorsing commercial products. No company wants its products associated with an athlete suspected of taking drugs.

Burwell believes that if testing must be done,

(Opposite page.) At the University of Nevada, head basketball coach Jerry Tarkanian instructs his team from the sidelines. Tarkanian supports drug testing.

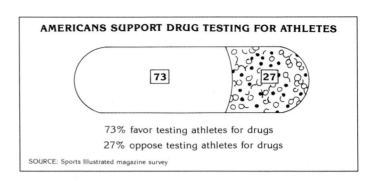

AMERICANS SUPPORT DRUG TESTING FOR ATHLETES

73% favor testing athletes for drugs

27% oppose testing athletes for drugs

SOURCE: Sports Illustrated magazine survey

tests should be conducted in a special facility where all the results would remain secret. Those testing positive would be counseled and given the necessary help they need to remain drug-free. If such a facility ever exists, it will benefit future players, but cannot help those players who have already suffered embarrassment and humiliation. Gene Upshaw, executive director of the NFL Players Association, agrees that a new system cannot repair the damage done to some players. "The real tragedy is that none of that will help any of these players. Their reputations have already been ruined. It's not fair," Upshaw says.

Being held to higher standards

The world of sports is divided between those who support drug testing of athletes and those who do not. While the debate rages on, drug testing continues. Regardless of the side he or she takes in the debate, nearly everyone agrees that, if it must be done, the testing should be accurate.

Those involved in drug-testing programs point out that a key factor in accurate testing is the element of surprise. In other words, athletes should not have plenty of advance notice of a test. Otherwise, they can stop taking drugs long enough for the substances to flush out of their systems. They will then test negative for drugs. Afterward, they can resume taking drugs and no one will be the wiser.

Several people, from both pro- and antitesting camps, are disappointed that some of the more common drugs are not even considered for drug testing. "Although studies have shown that alcohol and tobacco are the most abused drugs, no institution, including the NCAA [National Collegiate Athletic Association] and their list of three thousand banned drugs, tests for those two substances," Dr. Gary Green commented.

Athletes are role models

There is another important side to this drug-testing issue: whether or not athletes should be tested for drugs simply because they are athletes. Sports players make up one of the few social groups subjected to any kind of regular drug testing. Some people argue that because athletes have so much influence over other members of society, their behavior should be monitored. This includes testing them for drugs. William Bennett, director of the Office of National Drug Control Policy, said, "Athletes should be held to higher standards than other citizens."

Those opposed to Bennett's view believe that athletes should not have to live up to special standards. Though sports stars are in the public eye and looked up to by many, so too are actors, politicians, and Nobel Prize winners. Yet no one demands members of these groups be tested for drugs. One writer asked, "Why is the public so outraged when some quarterback or third baseman is picked up on a cocaine charge? When a John Belushi self-destructs, there is no outcry for the drug testing of actors. Outrage, it seems, is reserved for sports."

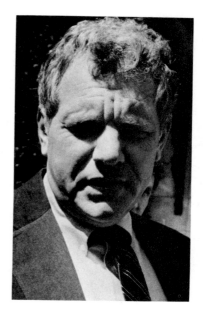

William Bennett, director of the Office of National Drug Control Policy, believes athletes should be monitored for drug use.

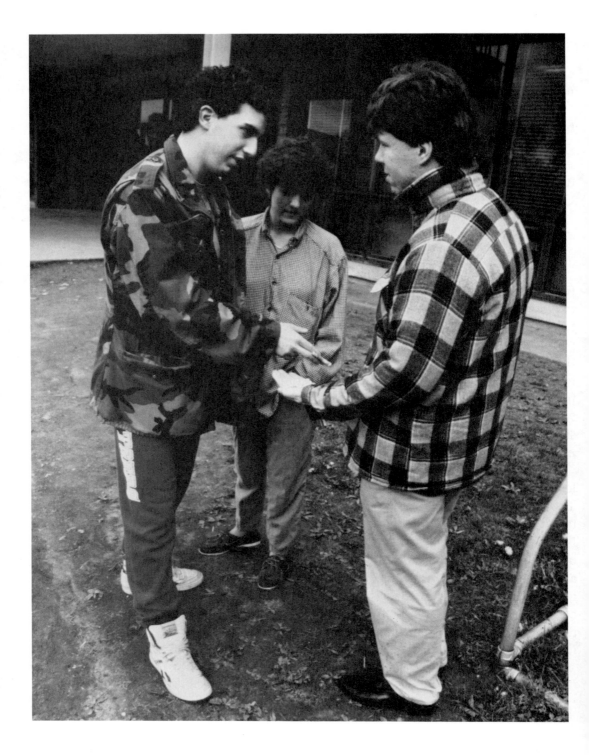

8

The Drugs and Sports Profiteers

FINANCIAL PROFIT is a major motivation for some people to get other people hooked on drugs. Both legal and illegal drugs are very big business, and the people who sell these drugs can make large profits. The alcohol and tobacco industries, for instance, gross billions of dollars a year each. The illegal steroids market is said to top $100 million a year. And untold billions are spent on other illegal drugs like cocaine and marijuana.

In the case of illegal substances like cocaine, there are many people who profit as use of the drug spreads. The most obvious profiteer is the dealer on the street. He or she is the one who makes new contacts and directly promotes the use of the drug. If the drug comes from another country, as is the case with cocaine, the people who smuggle the drug into the country also make a profit. In addition, those who grow and process the drug take their share. And, of course, the heads of drug rings, often called drug "lords" or "kingpins," take the biggest cut of the profits. It is in the interest of all these people to push their product and entice more people to become users; the more users there are, the more money the pushers make.

There are also several people and organizations that profit from the use of illegal steroids. The deal-

A drug dealer exchanges cocaine for cash. Selling illegal drugs can be very profitable for street dealers.

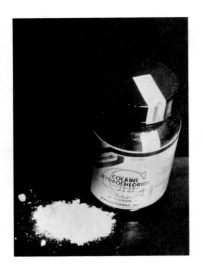

Billions of dollars are spent each year on cocaine, shown here in its powdered form.

ers at gyms and health clubs are the most visible steroid pushers. Their profits are considerable. One police investigator reported finding a dealer's gym bag that contained $170,000 in cash!

Because they turn large profits does not mean that steroid dealers are selective about the quality of their product. Many steroid dealers are careless about what they sell. Sometimes bottles are labeled incorrectly and customers get the wrong type of steroid. Other times, the drugs are "watered down" with cheap, nonsteroid substances. Occasionally, the customer does not get steroids at all. For example, one dealer bought bottles of vitamin B-12 at $2 a bottle and sold them as steroids for $150 a bottle. But these dealers are only part of the picture.

Drug companies illegal deals

Some large drug companies have made profits on steroids illegally. For instance, in the early 1980s, some companies that manufactured the drug for medical use secretly and illegally sold quantities of the substance to drug dealers. The dealers then went out and made their own profits selling the drug to members of the public. Eventually, the government stepped in and limited the amount of steroids the big companies could produce. That resulted in the establishment of many black market labs inside and outside the United States. These labs now supply most of the illegal steroids consumed by athletes as well as by the general public.

Other steroid profiteers are not so easily recognizable. That is because their immediate profits may not be in the form of cash. Yet they have something to gain from getting athletes to use steroids. For instance, coaches are often aware that players on their teams are taking steroids. In fact, some coaches have been known to personally promote and supervise the use of the drug. Sometimes a coach will get the team doctor to officially prescribe the drug. That way, the use of the drug is less likely to be questioned.

A coach might push steroid use by his or her players to gain personal prestige. If the team has a winning season, the coach will look good. Perhaps he or she will receive a salary raise or bonuses, or maybe favorable publicity will result. Some coaches, like some athletes, will do almost anything to win, including push illegal drugs.

Earlier, it was described how parents asked a doctor to use steroids to manipulate the growth cycles of their children. Such parents are as much a part of the illegal drug problem as the dealers on the street. While the street dealer is in it strictly for the money, the parent profits from a gain in prestige. For instance, a father may be admired by friends and associates if his son or daughter is a winning athlete. Because they influence others to unlawfully take drugs, these parents assume the role of the illegal drug pusher.

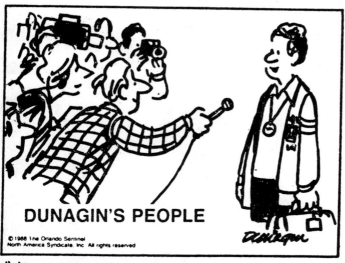

DUNAGIN'S PEOPLE

© 1988 The Orlando Sentinel
North America Syndicate, Inc. All rights reserved

"I'D LIKE TO THANK MY COACH, MY MANAGER, MY AGENT AND MY CHEMIST!"

The way the public views drug dealers depends on which drug is being promoted. When cocaine, nonprescription steroids, or other illegal drugs are involved, the issue of selling the drugs is usually clear-cut. The dealers are automatically labeled pushers and thought of as disreputable characters. They are subject to arrest, court trials, and imprisonment. On the other hand, consider the case of legal drugs like alcohol and nicotine. Here, those who promote the drugs are ordinary salespeople. They are often hard-working businesspeople, respected in the community and financially rewarded for their efforts.

Obviously, then, there is a double standard in the way society regards people who distribute drugs. Legal drugs are socially acceptable, so few people

A clerk sells alcohol to customers. Because alcohol is legal, its distribution is not regarded as disreputable.

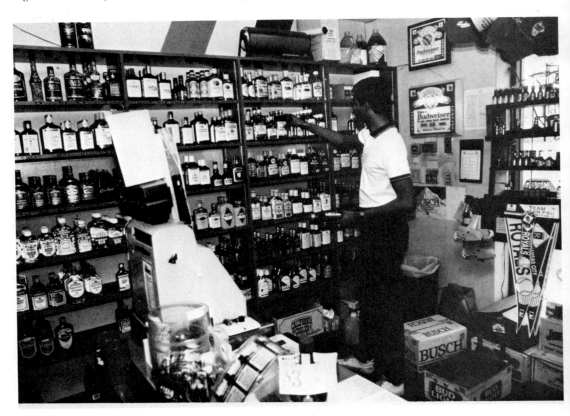

are upset when beer companies promote sporting events through sponsorship and advertising. The fact that a football game may be sponsored by a beer company establishes a relationship in the minds of the viewers—a link between alcohol and football. Each year, thousands of people are influenced to drink alcohol by such advertising. Some of these drinkers never experience any significant problems related to their alcohol use. But others eventually go on to become alcoholics with ruined lives. Yet almost no one blames beer companies or famous players for promoting the use of a dangerous drug. Instead, people who suffer from alcohol problems are themselves blamed, usually for being weak or self-indulgent.

Similar advertising promoting alcohol and link-

Advertisers promote the use of their products through sporting events. The name of a beer, Old Milwaukee, receives exposure at a racing event.

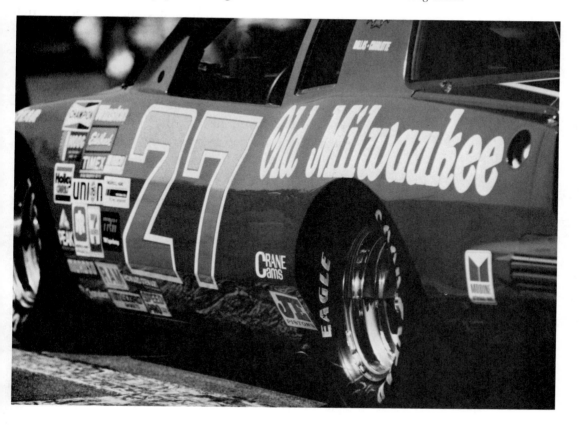

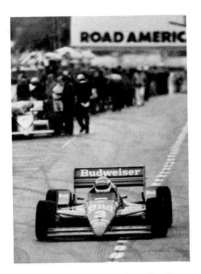

Budweiser beer is advertised at a race.

ing the drug with athletics appears in magazines and on billboards. In 1987, Anheuser-Busch, the largest beer company in the United States, spent $344 million on advertising. Two-thirds of this amount was devoted to sports-related areas.

Many people who work in alcohol-rehabilitation programs complain that they are fighting a losing battle. They say that the big alcoholic beverage companies can afford to spend far more convincing people to drink than drug counselors can to help people stop drinking.

Alcohol is not the only drug to have been widely promoted. Cigarettes used to be heavily advertised on television. Young, athletic models, along with well-known sports figures, such as golfer Arnold Palmer, extolled the virtues of smoking. Then, in the 1960s, the U.S. Surgeon General reported that smoking had been proven to be a serious health hazard. The medical community, antismoking groups, and insurance companies began to pressure legislators to limit tobacco advertising on television. Eventually, all cigarette ads were banned from television. However, newspaper, magazine, and billboard ads continue to recruit new smokers.

Cigarette ads make smoking look fun

Like the efforts of beer companies to sell their product, portrayals by tobacco companies of smoking are always upbeat. The ads try to associate smoking with vigorous outdoor types or well-to-do, fun-loving young adults. The only indication that the product is a drug with dangerous side effects is the health warning printed on cigarette packs on billboards, and in magazine ads. The government forced the tobacco companies to begin printing the warning in the 1970s. There is no evidence to show whether or not these reminders have had any effect on smokers.

The answer to the problem of eliminating illegal drugs may depend upon changing our attitudes toward legal drugs. As long as society sanctions the use of alcohol and nicotine, it may be difficult to convince people to avoid cocaine, marijuana, and other illegal drugs. Indeed, illegal drug users sometimes rationalize their drug abuse by pointing to widespread use of substances like beer and cigarettes. It might be that until we reevaluate our acceptance of legal drugs and change our habits, the problem of drug abuse in general will not go away.

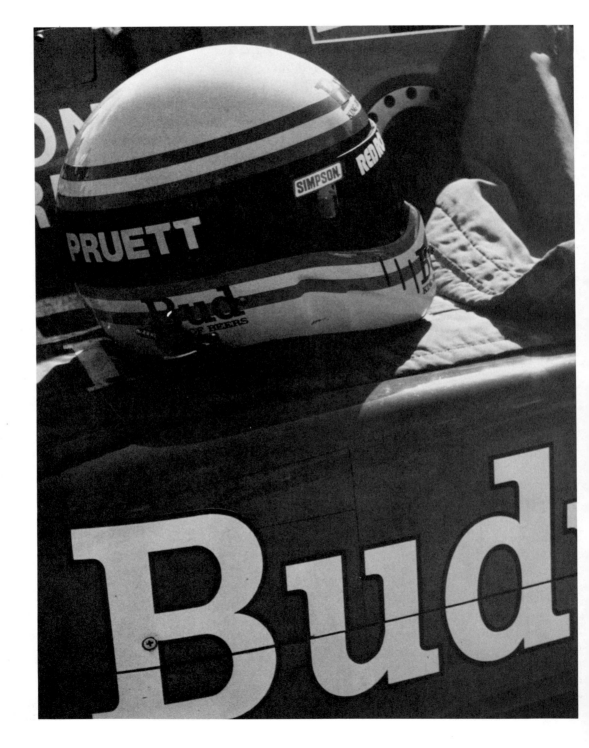

9

Fighting Drug Abuse in Sports

MANY U.S. drug officials see sports figures as having a special responsibility to help rid society of drug abuse. William Bennett said, "Professional sports plays a very important part in American life and a very important part in American imagination. Professional sports has to be part of the solution."

Speaking to leaders of major sports teams, Bennett repeated the belief that athletes are role models for young people. He also urged stricter penalties for players caught using illegal drugs. Many people agree with Bennett that famous athletes can and should set an example for nonathletes.

Sportswriter Rick Telander disagrees. He feels that the amount of influence athletes have on the behavior of nonathletes has not been clearly established. And, he argues, even if people in society do see athletes as major role models, it does not mean that athletes should be forced to behave in a certain way. Perhaps it is unfair to expect sports figures to set an example for everyone else. Gene Upshaw agrees: "We put athletes on so high a pedestal that we forget they're human."

But athletes are as human as everybody else, Telander argues. "The reasons some athletes take drugs," he says, "are the same reasons other adults

While companies such as Budweiser lend their names to promote a race, beer companies do not promote or condone drinking and driving.

do—stress, boredom, immaturity, depression, the quest for thrills." Telander believes that although some players are well-suited to be role models, imposing that burden on all athletes is unfair.

Some professional athletes who have willingly become role models have been especially effective in directing their peers away from drugs. Sam McDowell and Carl Eller are excellent examples. Both men suffered drug-related falls from the heights of sports fame and fortune. Both pieced their lives back together and became counselors for other players. And both men advocate the use of a new kind of peer pressure in athletics—the pressure *not* to use drugs. The theory behind such positive peer pressure is that if enough players on a team discourage any drug use they see, drug use by team members in general will decrease.

Coaches as role models

Hand-in-hand with the concept of athletes helping each other avoid drugs is the idea of coaches helping their players. A coach is in a natural position to act as a role model for team members. Many players, especially high school and college athletes, look up to coaches. To some, a coach can be a substitute parent. Team members often go to coaches for guidance off the field as well as on. Many sports figures feel that coaches should strictly enforce antidrug rules. This will create an atmosphere in which players will think twice about risking drug use. But those who favor this approach point out that actions speak louder than words. A coach should never say one thing and do another. For instance, a coach who smokes or chews tobacco while lecturing team members not to use drugs should not expect to be taken seriously. On the other hand, the coach who is seen to be totally drug-free might prove to be a positive role model for many players.

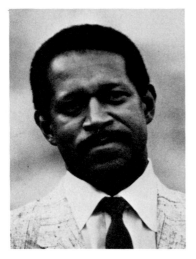

Gene Upshaw believes that the public should not impose exceptionally high standards on athletes. He maintains that drug use among athletes will stop only when it's halted in the general public.

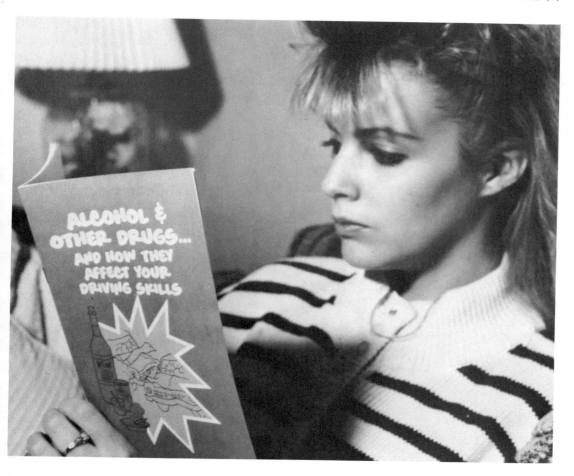

Most people who are concerned about drug abuse seem to agree that education is a major weapon in the war on drugs. Drug education takes many forms. Lectures, films, and class activities in schools, especially grade schools, have been one approach.

Another educational tool in the antidrug battle is media exposure of drug abuse. Newspapers, magazines, radio, and TV all increased the number and length of their antidrug messages in the 1980s. This exposure was partly responsible for a growth in public awareness about drugs in general. In particular, the media highlighted the problem of drinking and driving. As a result, many changes in alcohol-

A teenager reads an educational booklet that highlights the problems of drinking and driving.

related social habits occurred. For one thing, bars can be held liable for serving drinks to intoxicated patrons. Another significant change was a marked increase in the number of designated drivers, people who volunteer not to drink at parties and other functions where alcohol is served. These nondrinking volunteers safely drive home friends who have been drinking.

The antidrug media messages have often been delivered by well-known sports figures, such as Joe

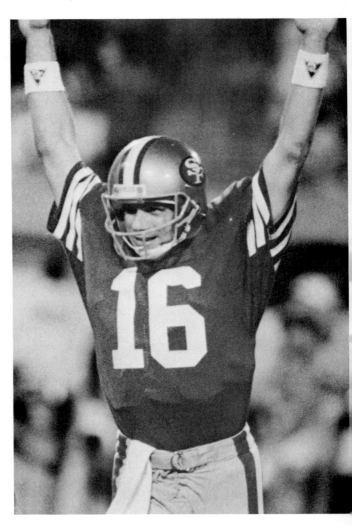

San Francisco 49ers quarterback Joe Montana raises his arms in victory after throwing a touchdown pass. Montana works with young athletes in an effort to prevent drug abuse.

Montana of the San Francisco 49ers. These athletes address everyone in society, but especially reach out to younger athletes. The messages emphasize that drugs will lower athletic performance levels as well as cause health problems or even death. Many prominent athletes including Jim Kelly of the Buffalo Bills, have toured schools, lecturing classes about drug abuse and chatting with young athletes on a one-to-one basis. The visiting players often suggest ways the school athletes can help prevent drug abuse.

They recommend, for example, "straight" parties, especially after games or meets. These parties, where only nonalcoholic beverages are served, remove the element of peer pressure to drink alcohol. Such parties also promote the idea that people can have a good time without getting drunk.

Visiting athletes also offer young players advice on how to cope with the stresses of training and competing. The players are taught how to effectively manage their time; to balance school and home duties with the demands of their chosen sports. They are also advised on ways to relax that do not involve drugs. These ways may include pursuing hobbies or getting involved in club activities.

Disagreements over testing and penalties

In addition to education, drug testing and law enforcement play important parts in the war on drugs. But testing remains highly controversial. Those who support testing sports players usually push for testing to begin early, on the junior high school level or even younger. The pro-test people say that fear of being caught is keeping many college and professional players from using drugs. Those who are against testing continue to insist that it invades the privacy of athletes. The antitest people

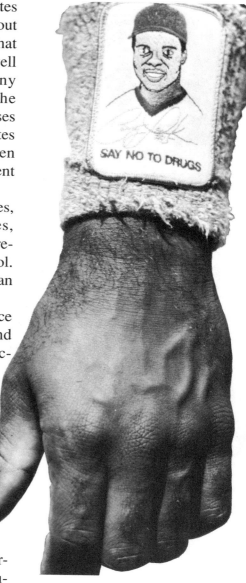

A sweatband with an antidrug message is used as a tool in the war on drugs.

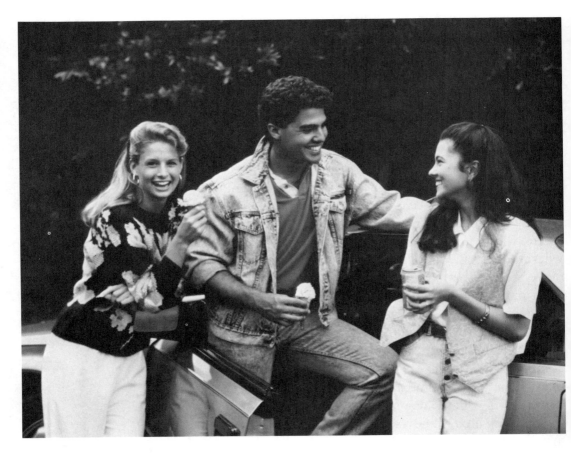

High school students share laughs while eating ice cream after school. The antidrug campaign is aimed at promoting a positive image of teens who say no to drugs.

say that the tests are not stopping athletes from taking drugs. Instead, players are just learning new ways to beat the tests.

Nearly everyone agrees that law enforcement officials on the federal, state, and local levels must continue to put every effort into the fight against illegal drug use. However, not everyone agrees on how the laws should be enforced. Many people think that penalties for drug abuse are too lenient, and some even think the death penalty should be given to drug pushers, especially drug kingpins. Others see the death penalty as ineffective in deterring the sale of illegal drugs. They also think that harsh penalties should be handed out only to big-time pushers, while penalties for users should be relaxed.

There are also heated arguments at all levels of government over just how much money should be allotted to fighting drugs. Some say more money will make a definite dent in illegal drug use. Others argue that more money is not needed, and that drug officials need to better manage the money they have.

The key to winning the war

Like drug abuse in society, drug abuse in sports will not go away by itself. All the antidrug tactics mentioned, from positive peer pressure and coaches acting as role models to media ads and law enforce-

Former Miami Dolphin great Mercury Morris (right) embraces Carl Eller after Morris's keynote address at the Cocaine Connection Conference.

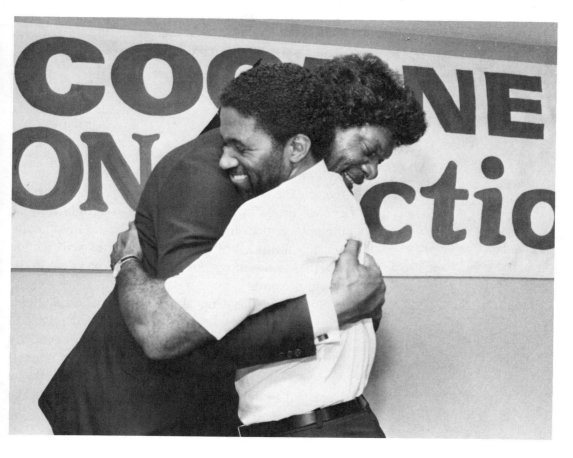

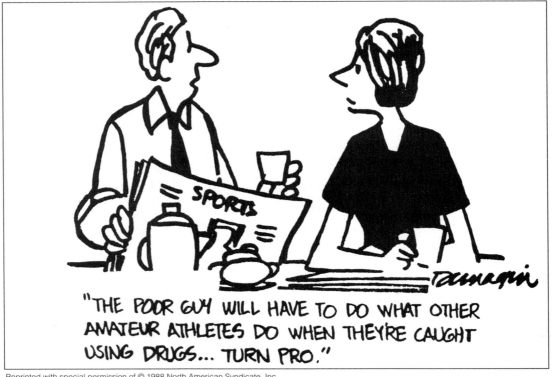

"THE POOR GUY WILL HAVE TO DO WHAT OTHER AMATEUR ATHLETES DO WHEN THEY'RE CAUGHT USING DRUGS... TURN PRO."

ment, will need to be used if the war on drugs is to be won. Each of these approaches will have an effect on the way players view drugs. Whether players see drugs in a positive or negative light may be the key element in the battle. For, in the final analysis, the attitudes of individual athletes will decide whether or not drugs continue to be a problem in the world of sports.

Some say the drug abuse situation is hopeless, that drugs will always plague society. Others recall the story of the lotus-eaters who were saved by Ulysses and take heart. Although Ulysses himself ate the flowers and felt their addictive effects, he managed to drag himself out of his stupor and save his crew as well as himself.

The ancient parable has its modern counterparts

in the stories of Carl Eller, Sam McDowell, and other courageous athletes. Offering strength and hope, they have shown that the most powerful force for fighting drug use is human beings helping each other.

Glossary

alcohol: A colorless liquid found in beer, wine, and liquor. The substance causes intoxication when consumed.

alcoholic: A person who is physically and/or psychologically addicted to alcohol.

alcoholism: A chronic disorder characterized by excessive drinking and dependence on alcohol.

amphetamines: Sometimes referred to as "speed"; stimulant drugs that make the user feel awake and alert.

anabolic: Having to do with the buildup of muscle tissue, as in anabolic steroids.

barbiturates: Sedative drugs that cause drowsiness. They are the main ingredient in many sleeping pills.

brake drugs: Drugs used to intentionally stunt the growth of athletes, especially female gymnasts.

caffeine: A stimulant found in coffee, tea, and colas.

cirrhosis: Severe scarring of liver tissue, usually as a result of alcohol abuse.

cocaine: An addictive stimulant drug derived from the coca plant.

crack: A pure form of cocaine. Crack can cause almost instant dependence.

depressant: A substance that acts to depress, or slow, the workings of the brain and nervous system.

drug addiction: Physical and/or psychological dependence on one or more drugs.

freebase: To heat cocaine to separate the cocaine base from other chemicals. The base is then smoked from a pipe.

hallucinogens: Drugs such as LSD and marijuana that can bring on hallucinations as a side effect.

hashish: Commonly referred to as "hash"; a potent, pastelike form of marijuana.

hormone: A substance manufactured in human cells that can have an effect on other body parts and functions; for instance, some hormones stimulate growth.

jaundice: Physical disorder in which the liver leaks toxic substances into the bloodstream.

marijuana: Commonly referred to as "grass"; a drug derived from the hemp plant that causes a feeling of well-being and drowsiness.

morphine: A powerful narcotic drug originally used by doctors to kill pain. It causes severe addiction in regular users.

nicotine: A highly addictive drug found in tobacco products.

performance-enhancing drugs: Drugs taken to improve strength, speed, or physical appearance.

recreational drugs: Drugs taken for personal pleasure.

sedatives: Drugs such as barbiturates that cause drowsiness.

smokeless tobacco: Tobacco that is chewed.

snuff: A powdered form of tobacco that is sniffed.

steroids: Drugs similar to or derived from testosterone. They are known to help build muscle mass and strength when used in small doses. Nicknames include "roid," "gas," and "juice."

stimulants: Drugs such as caffeine and amphetamines that make the user feel awake and alert.

strychnine: A poisonous substance sometimes taken in small doses to enhance athletic performance.

testosterone: A male hormone that controls secondary sex characteristics.

therapeutic drugs: Drugs prescribed by a doctor to help restore or maintain health.

tranquilizers: Sedative drugs used to calm anxiety.

Suggestions for Further Reading

Julie S. Bach, ed. *Drug Abuse, Opposing Viewpoints*. St. Paul: Greenhaven Press, 1988.

Virginia S. Cowart, "Athletes and Steroids—A Bad Bargain," *Saturday Evening Post*, April 1987.

Edward F. Dolan, *Drugs In Sports*. New York: Franklin Watts, 1986.

William Gildea, "Life—and Drugs—in Sports' Fast Lane," *Reader's Digest*, January 1988.

Gary Alan Green, "Drugs and the Athlete," *Delaware Medical Journal*, September 1987.

Mike Lupica, "The Alcohol Rub," *Esquire*, June 1988.

John Papanek, "Athletes or Role Models?" *Sports Illustrated*, June 15, 1987.

Rick Telander and T. Chaikin, "The Nightmare of Steroids," *Sports Illustrated*, October 24, 1988.

Paul Thompson, "Dope and Glory," *Runner's World*, December 1988.

Index

Picture Credits

Cover photo by: FPG, Bill Powers

Allsport, 6
American Cancer Society, 69, 71, 72
AP/Wide World Photos, 11, 13, 19, 46, 52, 61, 76, 85
John E. Biever, Third Coast Stock Source, 39
Simon Bruty, Allsport, 16
Paul C. Butterbrodt, Third Coast Stock Source, 94
D&I MacDonald, Third Coast Stock Source, 58, 59, 78
Patrick Dean, Third Coast Stock Source, 54
David L. Denemark, Third Coast Stock Source, 57, 63
Brian Drake, NMR, 53, 99
Thomas J. Edwards, Third Coast Stock Source, 20
Ed Gamble © 1986. Reprinted with permission, 79
Dave Gess, Third Coast Stock Source, 60
Jeff Greenberg, 86
Larry Hamill, 12, 80
Tim Haske, ProFiles West, 37
Ralf-Finn Hestoft, Third Coast Stock Source, 75
Robert Hitchman, Unicorn Stock Photos, 50
© Hofoss/Rothco. Reprinted with permission, 24
Cliff Hollis, ProFiles West, 41
Diane Johnson, Allsport, 96
King Features, North American Syndicate, Inc., 83, 89, 102
Caryn Levy, Allsport, 21, 36
P. Barry Levy, ProFiles West, 23
Howard Linton, Third Coast Stock Source, 22
Tom McCarthy, Unicorn Stock Photos, 100
MacDonald Photography, Third Coast Stock Source, 40, 88, 97
William Meyer, Third Coast Stock Source, 18, 27
Buck Miller, Third Coast Stock Source, 92
Ken Osburn, Third Coast Stock Source, 91
Mike Powell, Allsport, 25, 30
J. Rettaliata, Allsport, 62
Barry L. Runk from Grant Heilman, 9, 70
Allen Russell, ProFiles West, 34, 42, 44, 51
Grace Natoli Sheldon, Third Coast Stock Source, 73
Allen Dean Steele, Allsport, 47, 48, 49
Rick Stewart, Allsport, 65, 82
D. Strohmeyer, Allsport, 81
John Trever © 1983. Reprinted with permission, 74
David Tulis, UPI, 98
Unicorn Stock Photos, 38
United Features Syndicate, Inc., 33, 56
UPI/Bettmann Newsphotos, 28, 64, 101
Vandystadt, Allsport, 66
Aneal Vohra, Unicorn Stock Photos, 90

About the Author

Don Nardo is an actor, makeup artist, film director, composer, and teacher, as well as a writer. As an actor, he has appeared in more than fifty stage productions, including several Shakespeare plays. He has also worked before or behind the camera in twenty films. Several of his musical compositions, including a young person's version of H.G. Wells's *The War of the Worlds,* have been played by regional orchestras. Mr. Nardo's writing credits include short stories, articles, textbooks, screenplays, and several teleplays, including an episode of ABC's "Spenser: For Hire." In addition, his screenplay *The Bet* won an award from the Massachusetts Artists Foundation. Mr. Nardo lives with his wife and son on Cape Cod, Massachusetts.